INGREDIENT X

The Production of Effective Drugs

INGREDIENT X

The Production of Effective Drugs

by

Louis C. Schroeter, Ph.D.

Pharmaceutical Research and Development
The Upjohn Company, Kalamazoo, Michigan

PERGAMON PRESS

New York • Toronto • Oxford • London • Mexico City
Edinburgh • Sydney • Braunschweig • Buenos Aires

PERGAMON PRESS INC.
Maxwell House, Fairview Park, Elmsford, N.Y. 10523
PERGAMON OF CANADA LTD.
207 Queen's Quay West, Toronto 117, Ontario
PERGAMON PRESS LTD.
Headington Hill Hall, Oxford;
4 & 5 Fitzroy Square, London W. 1
PERGAMON PRESS S.A.
Villalongin 32, Mexico 5, D.F.
PERGAMON PRESS (SCOTLAND) LTD.
2 & 3 Teviot Place, Edinburgh 1
PERGAMON PRESS (AUST.) PTY. LTD.
Rushcutters Bay, Sydney, N.S.W.
VIEWEG & SOHN GmbH
Burgplatz 1, Braunschweig

Library of Congress Catalog Card No. 70-85147

Printed in United States of America

08 006862 6

Contents

Preface

INGREDIENT X tells about some of the exciting and challenging aspects of pharmaceutical research and development in simple, non-technical language. Over 50 illustrations are used to explain experiments and "tools of the trade". The importance of formulation ingredients on drug effectiveness is discussed in detail. Primary emphasis is placed on the pharmaceutical development scientist and his role in designing dosage forms for modern drugs. Pharmaceutical development is revealed as a challenging and rewarding career — the scientist encounters unusual opportunities to apply his broad knowledge of physical and biological sciences in the design of useful products. Translating research findings into products which restore health is a stimulating adventure in applied research. It is also a vitally important activity — effectiveness of today's drug product depends as much on the design of the formulation as it does on the drug itself.

CHAPTER I

Research And Development (R & D)

DEVELOPMENT

MAKING discoveries work is the exciting and challenging task called development — the D part of R & D. To apply the discovery, we must understand what the discovery is all about. Development involves the scientist in a continual learning process. This is one of the main reasons that it is so much fun. Development definitely is not easy — each problem is different. The measure of success, though, is always the same: the product must work. In other words, the development scientist plays in a most demanding game in which it matters very much whether the game is won or lost — playing well is not enough.

Speaking of games, development is a lot like the game of football — the scoring must be done in the allotted time. The assignment to develop a new kind of high potency vitamin formulation always involves a time limit. If it did not, the new product might be developed too late to fill the need, or, as often happens, someone else might develop it first.

Why the concern for being first? Simply this: the rewards in development are given in the same way as they are in games — to the first.

The very high cost of development is another reason for the concern about the time required to get the answer or to achieve results. If the cost to develop a new discovery is too high, the improved product may never pay for itself much less show a profit to those who made the discovery and carried out the development. The idea of setting a time limit on a development project begins to make sense when we consider development costs and the *expected* total return in profit on a new product. For example, if a new product is *expected* to show a total profit of $100 during its life on the market and, if the cost to develop it were $10 a day, development effort beyond 10 days or $100 total cost could hardly be justified from an economic standpoint. Sometimes this kind of "unprofitable" development may be carried out as a service to the medical profession to provide effective formulations of rarely used life-saving drugs.

The restrictions and limitations inherent in development activities make the job difficult. Nonetheless, the very nature of development provides a sense of the excitement found in few other kinds of research activity. The development project always involves clear-cut goals; achievement can be measured in terms of practicality of the results. Successful completion of an especially difficult development project provides a sense of great satisfaction to the scientist.

The main theme of this story deals with pharmaceutical product development — the kind of work done by the author. It is a vital and exciting adventure dealing with many aspects of science and technology. Hopefully, some of the fun and challenge will show through to the reader. Far too many books are written about what scientists do by people who have never done it. This is a story of a special kind of scientist who applies various elements of science and technology in his efforts to translate research findings into products. The products are of immense importance in that they are used to maintain or restore health. The effectiveness of today's drug products depends, in large measure, on the formulations developed by these scientists.

TWO KINDS OF RESEARCH

It is not the difficulty of the doing nor the person who does it that determines whether research is basic or applied. Intent and purpose of the research provide a good test. If the research is done mainly to increase knowledge of the world around us, it may be considered *basic*. If, however, the research has as its main purpose finding something useful to man in the immediate or near future, it may be considered *applied* research. But not all scientists agree with this definition. So, it is a good idea to find out just what is meant wherever the terms are encountered.

For example, a chemist may construct or synthesize a new compound having a very special structure for the purpose of determining its water solubility. The effect of molecular structure on solubility may be considered as basic or fundamental information about the physical world. When the experiment has been checked carefully, the chemist will publish the new information in a scientific journal so that others may verify it and use the data in their search for knowledge. Research that is done mainly to add to man's understanding of nature may be considered to be basic research. If the same chemist makes a gasoline additive compound, he is doing applied research in the sense that his knowledge is brought to bear or applied to solve a practical problem — the finding of an additive to improve gasoline performance. In the process of doing applied research, scientists also make many important contributions to basic knowledge. One thing can be said about the term applied research — no one readily agrees what it means, least of all, scientists. There is an unfortunate and unjustified tendency to look upon it as being less glamorous than basic research. A definition often used by scientists is: applied research is what others do; basic research is what I do!

TRAINING

The kind of work done by scientists will differ somewhat according to the degree or level of training. The student who successfully completes four or five years of university training receives a B.S. degree (Bachelor of Science); one to two years of advanced graduate training plus independent research work are required to qualify for an M.S. degree (Master of Science); three to four years of additional training beyond the M.S. plus successful completion of an independent research project (thesis) are required to qualify for the Ph.D. degree (Doctor of Philosophy). The extra training permits the scientist to start his career knowing more about his special area of interest. In general, scientists with advanced degrees will earn more money simply because they start their career in science with increased knowledge. This is not the main reason why scientists obtain advanced or graduate degrees. The real scientist — basic or applied — is driven by a desire to know and to understand. This is why he spends many years preparing for his life's work. His additional training rewards him many times over in added pleasure and deeper insights into problems encountered.

Academic degrees do not insure a lifetime of success. Far from it — they merely establish a certain level of competency or ability as of a certain date. In this respect, degrees are not like joining a club: the scientist must continue to study just to maintain a certain level of knowledge. It is hardly satisfying to stand still — most motivated persons will want to grow and achieve greater mastery of their field. In many respects, academic degrees are like the medals worn by soldiers in that they show evidence of achievement as of a certain date. Soldiers with many medals still continue to train for future battles and more difficult tasks. In the same way, scientists must continue to study and to learn.

For many years the training of scientists in the universities involved advanced study of specialized knowledge and a thesis problem for independent research. Now, as in the past, specialized knowledge is presented in courses of graduate instruction. The original research problem is conducted under the guidance of a professor who must evaluate the candidate's ability to do research. As might be expected, there is today *more* knowledge to master and the knowledge is more complex. The thesis problem involving original research or study on a specialized topic is expected to result in some new knowledge. In other words, it falls generally in the area of basic research. Today more research in the universities is being sponsored by governmental agencies to solve specific kinds of problems. That is, university research is becoming more applied. From a training point of view, this does not cause too much of a problem so long as the research program or study adheres to high standards of quality. The techniques of science are the same regardless of the purpose of the study. The danger of pursuing applied research in the university is that other important areas of investigation may be neglected in favor of the "popular" or more rewarding projects.

The problems encountered in the laboratory will more than likely determine whether or not a scientist spends most of his time doing basic or applied research. This is true even in applied research laboratories. The problem of preventing apple slices from browning serves as a good example of this. The scientist given this task might be trained in biological chemistry. Very likely his university training would provide him with some basic knowledge and background information related to the problem. All of his experience with apples may have been confined to eating them. The scientist's basic knowledge about the browning process would serve as a starting point in the project. Knowing something about the mechanism of the browning phenomenon puts the search for a way to prevent it on a sound basis. A rational approach would be based on the information that oxygen is involved and that trace amounts of metals make the browning reaction go faster. If available knowledge about the process of browning proved to be inadequate, it would have to be studied in sufficient depth before a way to prevent it could be found. The scientist working on the problem would, at various stages, be involved in both basic and applied science.

Utility or usefulness of results is a distinguishing mark of applied research. In some way, man benefits directly, and this benefit comes in a relatively short time. The problems applied scientists solve generally are as difficult as the problems encountered in basic research, differing mainly in that there is some element of immediate utility in the solution. Another point that is particularly challenging about applied research is that success can be measured against expectations. For example, if the problem is to find a way of preserving ready-sliced apples so that they will not turn brown, there is an objective way of evaluating proposed solutions. Usefulness of a new preservative can be tested against the performance of other preservatives under identical conditions. There is no substitute for results!

Another aspect of applied research is that the acceptable solution may be limited by a number of requirements that may conflict in whole or in part. The ultimate solution may have to be a balance between various factors. For example, discovery of a chemical that would prevent browning of apple slices would be worthless if this chemical were harmful to man. Likewise, the cost of the solution to the problem must be realistic. Not many people would use a preservative for apples that costs more than the apples! A preservative that would be both safe and cheap would not be acceptable if it altered the taste or color of the apples. Applied research is exceptionally demanding because acceptable solutions to problems must be found within a framework of many limiting factors.

"INERT" INGREDIENTS

Each successful pharmaceutical product contains, in addition to the active ingredients, one or more ingredients specially selected and present in some definite concentration. The special ingredients — we will call them all ingredient "X" — are selected very carefully with an eye toward making the most effective product. It is not enough to know that an ingredient is effective in the formulation. Knowing *why* ingredient X "works" permits the development scientist to select other ingredients for future improvement or for use in similar formulas. The search for the reason "why" brings the development scientist back to basic research and completes the circle of research-to-development and back to research. The process of defining the problem in this way helps to focus attention on areas of important study for the basic research group.

Additives or so-called "inert" ingredients may greatly affect the performance of the active or drug components in tablets or other kinds of dosage forms. The physical form in which the dose of the drug is prepared is known as the *dosage form*. Familiar dosage forms include tablets, capsules, syrups, injectables, and ointments. The dosage form is a complex system for protecting the drug and making it easy to take. More than this, it is a system for delivering a drug to the site of absorption in the body in an effective and reliable manner.

There can be significant differences in the effectiveness of different tablet formulations each containing the *same* weight or amount of the *same* drug. The "inert" ingredients are not really inert — the amount and kind affect the way the product performs. Each such ingredient might be considered to be an X-type additive. The idea of performance of a drug tablet might be grasped better by considering the performance of automobiles. It is hardly meaningful to compare two automobiles on the basis of the weight of steel they contain. This notion of equivalence seems far-fetched when applied to machinery, but it is often erroneously applied to dosage forms. Actually, the factors affecting performance of a dosage form like a tablet are every bit as varied and complex as those affecting machine performance.

A tablet containing 5 grains of aspirin will weigh a good bit more than the listed drug content. The added weight is due to the presence of additives needed to make the drug into a tablet and to ensure that the tablet releases the drug when it is taken by the patient. The ratio of additive to drug varies according to drug properties and other factors. A tablet containing 100 milligrams (mg.) of drug A might have a total weight of 400 mg. Making a tablet containing 200 mg. of the same drug would then seem to require 600 mg. of additives to give a tablet weighing 800 mg. Actually, this would be a pretty big tablet and not especially easy to take. This is a typical problem in which the development scientist must balance factors of additive effectiveness and tablet size. To do this successfully, it is necessary to carry out appropriate laboratory and clinical tests to make certain that the tablets behave in the same way even though the ratio of drug to additives may have been changed.

Flavor of a product often is a determining factor in its continued popularity. This is especially true of medicine to be taken regularly. For antacid tablets designed to be chewed rather than swallowed, the taste should be as good as possible. The taste also must remain good after prolonged storage. Changing the package from a tightly closed glass container to a plastic package offers one solution and, with it, a big problem. Some plastic bottles permit loss of flavor from the tablets. Revising the formula would then require an added "new" ingredient: the same flavor in a form that does not leave the tablet so readily. The identifying flavor of the product could, in one sense, be considered an inert ingredient but it isn't really — it is vital to the success of the product. In this respect, flavors, too, qualify as ingredient Xs.

Another example of an X-type ingredient is the antioxidant added to prevent oxygen from destroying vitamin A in certain multivitamin formulations. Without this "inert" ingredient, the vitamin preparations would not possess a long shelf life. A high quality formula stabilized with small amounts of a safe antioxidant may retain full potency for as long as 36 months. Another formula containing the same amounts of vitamins but no antioxidant would retain its potency for only 12 months. The consumer does not get full value if he purchased the unstabilized preparation. Another problem is encountered even if the preparation has an expiration dating of 12 months — it is a question of economics. The expired, short-dated product must be returned and more manufactured to replace it. The ultimate effect is increased cost to the consumer. Vitamin products containing an antioxidant ingredient clearly provide important advantages.

Availability of the drug from the dosage form is one of the most important performance factors to be considered in pharmaceutical product designing. We must be absolutely certain that the drug is released from the dosage form so that it is available for physiological absorption. This is an essential requirement! In the case of a tablet formulation, each and every tablet must contain the same amount of drug and it must release that drug in an absolutely reliable and reproducible fashion. Adding surfactant or wetting agent to a tablet or capsule formulation may so greatly improve drug absorption that the dose might be reduced from, say, 300 mg. to 200 mg. The wetting agent, added in low concentration, would indeed be an X-type ingredient.

Drug performance may be increased by controlling the way in which the drug is made available for absorption from the dosage form. In addition to possible therapeutic advantages, the prolonged release of drug from a dosage form may permit a change in the dosing schedule. The patient appreciates the convenience of prolonged release when it results in once-a-day rather than three-times-a-day dosage. Accomplishing this drug release pattern might require several "inert" ingredients. Considerable technology or know-how must be used in combining or using additives in the formula to achieve the desired effect. Controlling the rate at which drug is made available to the body for absorption represents a significant scientific accomplishment. Designing such systems to give predictable duration of drug action expands the usefulness of known and established drugs.

UTILITY

Product development also involves looking at old things in new ways. A drug of long standing used for treating the symptoms of hayfever or colds might be marketed by a number of different companies in the form of tablets, capsules, and fluid products. A new formulation might be devised that would use the same "old" drug in a new and *useful* way. By coating small granules of the drug so that the drug is released from a tablet over a long period, it may be possible to prolong the action of the drug. The "old" drug, in this new prolonged release form, would possess a distinct advantage if one such tablet could give relief through the night. The utility or usefulness of the new formulation is an important aspect of the development scientist's contribution. Success of the new product is judged by consumer acceptance — this is decided on the basis of value to the user.

Benefits to the consumer form the lasting basis for the successful product. Extensive advertising might effectively bring a product to the attention of a lot of people. If the product does not provide genuine benefits, no amount of advertising can provide sustained consumer acceptance. A good-tasting antacid product that does not perform as well as others in relieving symptoms of stomach distress likely will not be purchased a second time. Good taste is a desirable feature, but not the main reason why an antacid is purchased. The user expects the product to provide some relief from his distress — this is the measure of product performance.

The development scientist must keep always in mind what function the product is to perform and how it will be judged by the user. A drug product might be designed that would have a long storage life, say, five years, but would not taste good nor perform as effectively as other comparable products. The long shelf life might qualify as a significant scientific accomplishment. The product, however, would likely be judged a development failure by consumers because they received no perceptible benefits.

THE BIG CAKE BAKE

Scaling-up a process is always a special challenge for the development scientist. It is much like the problem involved in baking one cake in a home oven and then trying to write a recipe for making 1,000 cakes. One solution is to make one thousand individual cakes. This, of course, is hardly "Practical" — a favorite word of development scientists.

Making one thousand cakes from a single mix involves a great deal more than multiplying quantities of ingredients by a factor of 1,000 and then following the same directions. The order of mixing and combining the ingredients might have to be changed; even the amounts of ingredients may need altering to give a cake with the same taste and texture. The time for baking and the temperature of baking would likely be different. The critical test, after all, is that the cake made from the large recipe tastes the same as the one made from the individual mix. The same is true of pharmaceutical formulas: the product made on a large scale must have the same quality as the one made in the laboratory.

Development always involves details. Many variable factors must be balanced in the scale-up operation to obtain the best yield of high quality product. The development scientist's efforts may make the difference between profitable and non-profitable operations. This, in turn, may decide whether or not a company engaged in a highly competitive market is able to remain in business. Ultimately, this is related to jobs for workers! The development scientist plays a vital role in the success of technology-based companies.

A KEY FACTOR

Planning is one of the key factors in the success of a product development project. Developing a successful pharmaceutical product is a complex operation. It must be accomplished within a fixed time span and at costs compatible with anticipated returns. While this objective is always clearly in sight, simply saying that our goal is a successful product tells little about the exacting and challenging effort involved in balancing the many critical factors.

Taking stock of the situation is one of the first things that a development scientist must do at the start of a project. In this respect, he is like a battle commander: he must find out the relative strengths and weaknesses in his knowledge about the project and he must evaluate the resources available to achieve success. First of all, he might find out what the problem is or, more commonly, what the problems are. Each development project — like each battle — is different and yet there are similarities. There is a kind of order of battle associated with each development project in which plans are made and timetables drawn up. For a drug previously available only as a capsule, the following development timetable would apply for the design and evaluation of a tablet dosage form:

(1) Measure the rate of drug release from capsules. (1 week)

(2) Formulate the drug into prototype or experimental tablet formulations. (2 weeks)

(3) Measure the rate of drug release from the several tablet formulas and pick the one closest to that found for capsules for further development. (1 week)

(4) Reformulate the tablet to obtain drug release as close to that of capsules as possible. (2 weeks)

(5) Make larger batches of the tablets. (1 week)

(6) Check if drug release is same from larger lot sizes. (1 week)

(7) Put tablets on accelerated shelf life testing program (more about this later). (4 weeks)

(8) Determine if uniform tablets can be made from different samples of drug and other formulation components. (4 weeks)

(9) Check tablet stability in different types of containers. (4 weeks)

(10) Prepare tablet formula for safety testing in animals. (2 weeks)

(11) Prepare tablets for clinical testing. Compare results with those obtained in same subjects using capsules. (8 weeks)

(12) Carry out scale-up studies and evaluate effect of long term normal storage conditions. (52 weeks)

This schedule of 82 weeks to obtain a final tablet formulation does not include all of the time involved in testing of the dosage form. A considerable amount of laboratory and clinical testing of the final formula must be carried out. Safety and effectiveness must be proven before the drug may be marketed under a government-approved New Drug Application.

Defining the problem and then sketching out pathways that might be followed is a part of the planning that is done on development projects. Looking at all the problems that need solving can be a bewildering experience. It is far better to list those that should be solved in order of importance — a first things first kind of list. Then we must consider *how* this will be done and *what* information is needed. For example, we might have the problem of making a tablet containing two drugs which react when mixed together. This problem might be approached in the following way:

SITUATION REPORT	*OBJECTIVE*
When mixed, DRUG A + DRUG B react to lose potency.	Make a single solid dosage form containing DRUG A + DRUG B that does not lose potency and is fully effective.

Pathways that might be followed to achieve the objective:

1. Coat Drug A → Mix with Drug B → Make Capsules → Test Stability
   → Coat Drug B

   Mix Coated A with Coated B → Make Capsules → Test Stability

2. Make Pill of Drug A → Coat Pill of Drug A

   Put Pill into Capsule with Powder Drug B → Test Stability

Many more pathways can be written. In each, we would have the same elements: where we are, where we want to go, and how we propose to get there.

Almost all objectives can be met so long as there is enough time to pursue all the pathways that can be devised using available basic knowledge. When we come to the limits of present science and technology, the frontiers must be explored and expanded to provide the needed information. Recognizing this, there is always a great temptation to do one more experiment and to try one more pathway before giving up. The boundless enthusiasm and natural optimism of the scientist makes it easy to keep trying no matter how long it takes. It is at this point that the development scientist must exercise his best technical judgment to decide whether or not the project should be continued. Information needed to solve the critical problems may take additional months or even years to make the development objective even remotely possible — this can be an enormously expensive process. The cost of acquiring added data must be balanced against the expected profits that must ultimately result from the project. Profits are always a matter of concern to the development scientist — costly R & D expenses are paid for out of profits resulting from the sale of products.

Developing a product according to plan requires, first of all, an operating philosophy: the product should be effective and yet as simple as possible! Simplicity of product design means that the additive components should be as few in number as possible and used in optimum or best concentrations. Knowing *why* each ingredient is present in the formula and *why* it is present in the specified amount is essential to this concept of formulation. The optimum amount of an X-type ingredient may be arrived at on the basis of prior scientific knowledge. Often it is determined experimentally by trying different levels of ingredients in the formula and measuring over-all effectiveness.

In some formulas there may be more than one active ingredient and a large number of "inactive" ingredients — the concentration of which must be optimized. The problem of optimizing just one ingredient may involve tens or even hundreds of experiments. This is a time-consuming process. Time is always a limiting factor to the development scientist's efforts. The supply of time is fixed — it must be spent wisely and well. Each experiment must be designed to provide the maximum information in the minimum time.

Planning involves the assignment of an order of importance to each of the development operations. The plan must be reviewed in the same manner that a house under construction is inspected at various stages. This is done to make certain that the total effect of quality is achieved. In house building, the walls are not plastered until the wiring is properly done. Similarly, a fluid preparation would not be flavored until it had been established that the drug is reasonably stable in the unflavored system. By considering the time necessary to study the various factors in a project, and the order in which these should be performed, it is possible to construct

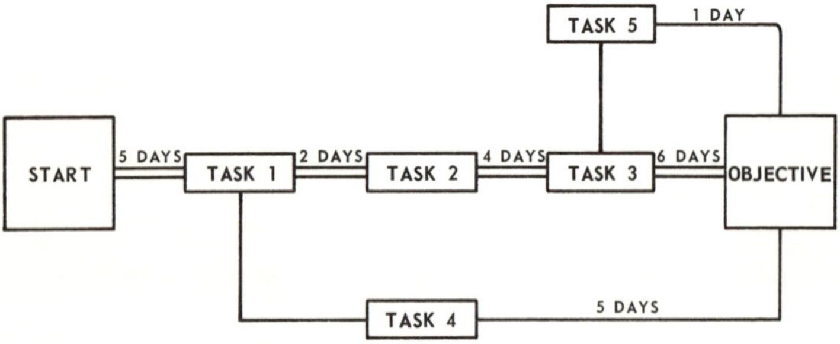

FIG. 1. Critical path schedule for development projects.

a critical path schedule. This is a pathway describing those tasks that would be hold-ups or rate-determining steps in the overall achievement of the objcetive.

The critical path shown here as a double line requires 17 days to complete. The value of such a scheme is that it points out where major effort should be directed to shorten the time span. A maximum effort to complete Task 4 in half the scheduled time would have no effect on overall time required. In other words, Task 4 is not on the critical path.

BALANCING ACT

The new pharmaceutical product must measure up to a number of rather stringent requirements. The point that the product must be acceptable to the consumer is easily understood as is the requirement that it maintain its quality on storage. The new product also must be capable of being

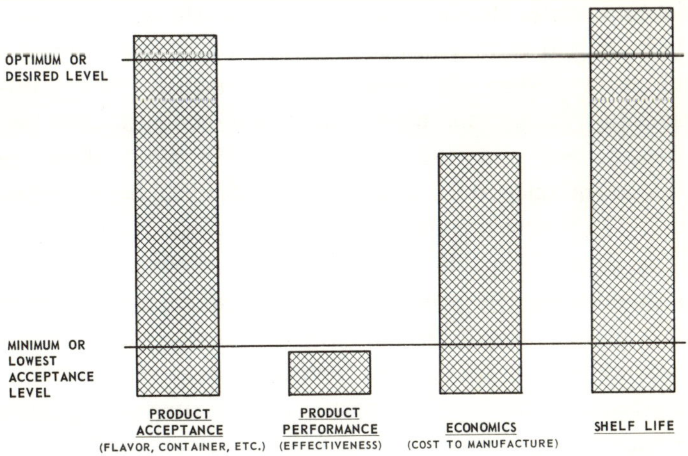

FIG. 2. Essential factors in the design of a new drug product.

manufactured at a reasonable price if the benefits are to be available to the largest number of people. The requirements for a successful product are not always completely compatible — the development scientist must balance a number of factors to obtain a product having the best possible combination. At various times during the development of a new product, the experimental formulations must be evaluated. This involves a systematic comparison of factors affecting product success. The profile of an experimental dosage form might appear as diagrammed in Figure 2 to the development scientist.

A formulation exhibiting such a profile would be judged a poor product candidate. High ratings in one or more categories are not sufficient to overcome a deficiency in the all-important factor of product effectiveness.

Perhaps the most fascinating part of development operations is the way that the projects increase in scope and grow in complexity. Because our scientific knowledge is constantly increasing, the development scientist must design products to meet higher standards of performance. The factors affecting quality are more varied and complex each year. Benefits and costs are constantly in the mind of the development scientist as he considers balancing the many factors which influence the success of a project. He knows that it is always desirable to have the new product provide the maximum possible benefits. It is also important to remember that development costs will increase sharply with increasing product performance goals. Development is very much like a picture puzzle to which pieces are constantly being added. Standards of product quality go ever upward and the task of balancing the many factors becomes a greater challenge with each new project. The development job never becomes routine no matter how many projects have been successfully completed in the past.

GROWING OLD

All products — even the best — grow old in time. This process of obsolescence is caused by man's ever-increasing knowledge and not by a fault in the initial product design. Mechanical and electronic devices suffer from obsolescence and so do drug formulations. Automobiles provide a familiar example of machinery that quickly becomes obsolete. Look at a 10-year-old car — not an old, worn-out one, but one in top condition. The old car simply does not have the performance and safety features of a new model. An automobile museum provides a vivid illustration of the way machinery goes out of date and is supplanted by newer, improved models. This is the kind of obsolescence that is easy to see — the outside appearance of cars changes with every model.

One notable exception to the practice of changing outside appearances is the popular German automobile, the Volkswagen. This beetle-shaped car has remained essentially the same on the outside but, over the years, has constantly changed on the inside. Its performance has been improved and, in this way, the dreaded obsolescence has been avoided. Many of the older, established drugs are in this way similar to the Volkswagen — the outward appearances have remained unchanged but the inner workings of the dosage form have been improved. The familiar aspirin tablet has contained 5 grains of aspirin for many, many years. The amounts and kinds of additives used in the aspirin tablets have changed and so has the performance. Some of the changes have involved processing improvements and better storage properties, but the most significant change has been in the speed with which the drug is absorbed to cure a headache. That is what performance is all about — the product does what it's supposed to do.

After the development scientist has designed a product incorporating the best possible balance of factors, the product is introduced to the consumer. In the case of a proprietary drug, it will be promoted directly to the public. Prescription drugs are promoted to physicians since they may be used only on their written order. It is interesting to look at the history of a product which incorporated the best know-how at the time of its introduction. Typically, the sales of the product increase to a high point during its introduction. This level is maintained for a time and then undergoes a steady decline as shown in Figure 3.

Why should there be a decline? In a free and competitive market, other pharmaceutical firms may, if they so choose, introduce their top candidate. The new product must not only compete against products on the market at the time it is introduced, but also against the best entries of other firms introduced at later times. In this way, the consumer has the best product that modern science and technology can offer. Even when the product contains an old, established drug, the user wants to be certain that the dosage form releases the drug in the most effective, reliable fashion and that the *highest* standards of present-day science are used to design and make the product. No one is satisfied with yesterday's best!

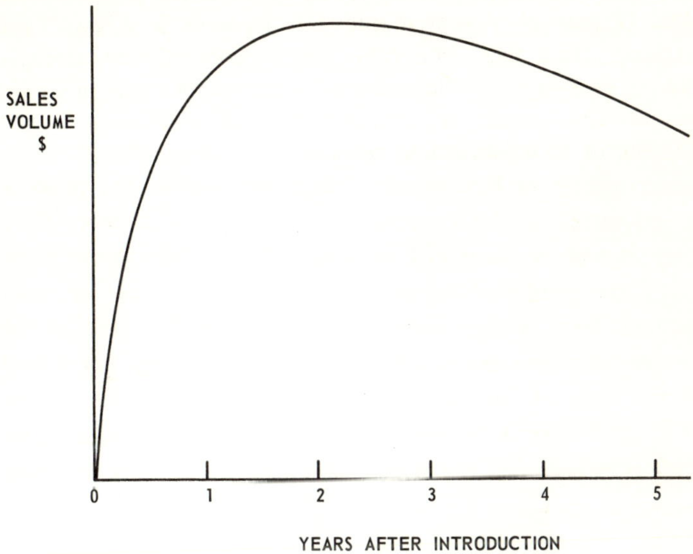

FIG. 3. Sales history of a new drug product.

TACTICS AND STRATEGY

The product development scientist must be an able strategist. He must make plans that take into account all of the important factors involved in designing superior products. The products must provide real benefits and must prove profitable. He must understand the complex ideas of modern science and technology. Comprehension of knowledge or even creation of concepts is not enough — the planning must be put into action. A scientist working in basic areas of science may comfortably stop at the point of introducing a new theory and be hailed a success. Not so with the development scientist — his efforts must result in useful products or processes. The D part of Research and Development is a great and exciting game that, like other highly competitive games, is always changing. Development is for the intellectually able and emotionally tough. It provides limitless challenges and a lifetime of stimulation and reward.

CHAPTER II

Product Acceptability

FROM TINCTURES TO TABLETS

ICEBOXES are but a memory and kerosene lamps a curiosity from the past — both victims of the rapid pace of technological advancement. The acceptable products of yesteryear are of interest to collectors, not to consumers. Product acceptability is redefined each day. People select for their use those products which best fill their needs and give the most — quality and quantity — for their money. Product acceptability is decided by the user and *not* by the maker. A new product may represent a great technical accomplishment and yet meet with little consumer support. The product must have qualities that consumers want. The product development scientist must design products with this thought clearly in mind. Often the quality appealing most to the user is achieved by adding just the right amount of some "inert" ingredient — a factor X.

The problem of lighting our way in the night or storing food has been with us a long time. In this century, such marvelous inventions as the electric light bulb and the mechanical refrigerator have filled a real need and have been developed to a high degree of efficiency and reliability. Although not as well recognized, similar progress has been made with drug formulations. Acceptability and effectiveness of tablets and other dosage forms have been improved in very significant ways. Perhaps you might think that the improvements are too complex to be easily understood. Certainly they are not so apparent as looking at the difference in brightness between a kerosene lamp and an electric bulb. To make matters worse, understanding is often obscured by the special jargon used by experts in describing these unique products. We will look at the changing patterns of product acceptability in simple, straightforward language.

Convenience to the consumer is a matter of great importance. Each new product must pass this test and must continue to meet it. Pharmaceutical products are no exception to the rule! Years ago, most of the drugs were natural materials or products derived from medicinal plants. Leaves and other parts of the medicinal plant were ground into a powder which was then steeped in hot water to extract the active drug constituent. The resultant fluid product was called an infusion; it had an advantage in that it could be taken in measured doses. Infusions made from fresh, fully active drug plants were reasonably effective. These preparations had one big disadvantage: they were not very convenient. An added problem was the extreme variability in potency and the tendency to spoil. Patients taking a digitalis infusion for the treatment of a heart condition had to have this medicine freshly prepared every few days at the pharmacy. If the infusion were stored over a week, it tended to lose potency. It also spoiled quite readily. Look at a three-day-old cup of tea. This will give you some idea of the spoilage problem!

Uniformity of dose was an enormous problem with drugs extracted from medicinal plants by the infusion process. Drug content of the plants varied according to the time of year and with age. To make matters worse, slight changes in the extraction procedure such as temperature of the water or time of exposure would result in great changes in the potency of the product. Sometimes these variables might cancel each other and a product of proper potency would result. More often, the variables would not cancel each other. The result would be extremely wide and often dangerous variations in potency of the product.

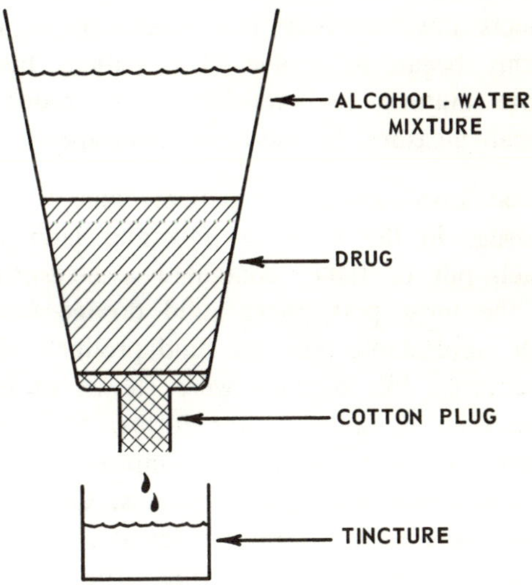

FIG. 4. Preparing a drug tincture by percolation.

The variable dose problem with drugs derived from medicinal plants prompted the introduction of tinctures. These are fluid preparations made by extracting the active ingredients from the finely powdered drug with an alcohol-water mixture. The powdered drug plant was moistened with an alcohol-water mixture and then packed into a funnel-like device called a percolator (see Fig. 4).

The drug was allowed to stand in contact with the fluid. After 24 hours standing, the fluid was allowed to drip or percolate slowly into a container. Due to the presence of alcohol, tinctures proved to be more resistant to spoilage than were infusions of the same drug. Furthermore, tinctures of potent drugs like digitalis were standardized in potency and maintained their drug activity during storage. Dosages of potent tinctures could be accurately measured in drops. These early fluid products illustrate how new standards of quality for dosage forms began to evolve. The patient benefitted by having more uniform and reliable drug products — and, in some small measure, by increased convenience.

An added advantage to the patient came with individual doses of drugs in the form of pills and later compressed tablets. Each pill or tablet contained a measured dose of drug. For the most part, these solid dosage forms proved to be much more stable than the fluid products of the same drug. Some drugs like digitalis were shown to be sensitive to moisture even in solid dosage forms. Problems of this sort prompted extensive efforts to improve the containers used for moisture-sensitive drug products. One of the more successful of these early designs employed a chemical drying agent (calcium oxide) to protect the drug from moisture. The drying agent was added to the bottom of the container and separated from contact with the dosage forms by a wad of cotton.

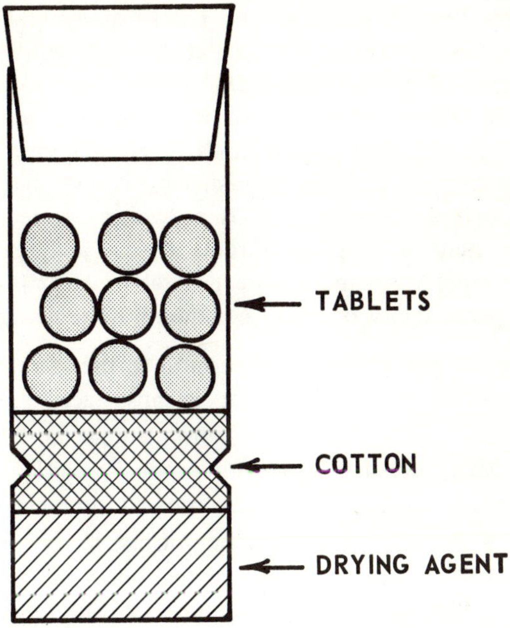

FIG. 5. A special bottle for protecting tablets from moisture.

POROUS BOTTLES

The first glass containers were stoppered with corks. Later, plastic screw caps were used because this permitted easier resealing and gave better protection. In time, plastics became available for use as containers. Initially, plastic containers found consumer acceptance for products other than pharmaceuticals. But, the sign was clear — they would, in time, find increasing consumer favor for all products including drugs. Plastic containers proved desirable because they were lighter than glass and not so easily broken. There were, however, some problems encountered with the use of early types of plastic containers. All of the problems have not been solved — many are being studied today. Fluid products packaged in certain kinds of plastics may lose volatile flavoring or perfume ingredients. Permeability of such plastics to volatile substances is a two-way street. The formulation may pick up undesirable flavors and odors if improperly stored. Another, more general problem involves the oxygen permeability of many commonly used plastics.

Since oxygen of the air is harmful to the storage qualities of most drugs, the development scientist faced a real challenge when packaging certain formulations in plastic containers. Many old and successful products which were completely stable in glass containers proved unstable in plastic containers. A trade-off or balancing of one factor — consumer preference — against economics or feasibility had to be made. Enormous difficulties were encountered with some formulations. Stabilizing the formula with additives (ingredient Xs) proved to be successful in most cases. For some sensitive products, packaging in plastic containers was not possible until better kinds of plastic became available. Achievement of pharmaceutical development objectives may be adversely affected by gaps in related sciences or technologies. The development scientist continually encounters the problem of extending projects beyond the available knowledge. It is always wise to have development operations backed up by sound basic information. The greatest challenge comes in trying to decide whether to stop the project and wait for basic science to catch up or to divert resources and find the necessary fundamental information. The last choice is not always easy even if it holds the promise of being first — it may require prohibitive amounts of time, talent, and money and still not give a pay-off. Knowing when to hold fast and when to advance is as important in research and development as it is in warfare. Success or failure is strongly dependent on making the right move at the right time.

HOW SWEET IT IS OR WHO DECIDES THE TASTE

Consumer preference has played a role in determining the flavor of medicines. Not too many years ago, it was generally accepted that medicine should taste bad. The "wonder" drugs of those days were usually the active constituents of medical plants. Almost all of these vegetable drugs were extremely bitter. Since the patient accepted the idea that medicine tasted bad, the notion grew that drug effectiveness was related to bad taste. As luck would have it, most of the newer synthetic drugs and antibiotics taste just as bad as the old drugs obtained from medicinal plants. In the meantime, peoples' ideas about the taste of medicines had changed. The idea caught on that being sick is unpleasant enough without having to take bad tasting medicine. The desire to have the product taste as *good* as possible must be balanced against other factors. It would hardly benefit the patient to make a product taste like chocolate candy if it did not release the drug when taken.

Who decides the taste of a new product? Initially, it is decided by the development scientist who makes it. Of course, the people who use the product are the ones who finally decide if the taste is good! In deciding whether or not to accept the product, taste evaluation always plays a part. The development scientist should know something about flavor preferences of people — big and little. If the product is sold on a world-wide basis, it is also important that he knows something about flavor preferences of people in other lands.

Flavor preferences change as people get older. This presents a problem for the development scientist who relies solely on his own or other adult taste preferences when flavoring a product for use by children. One solution to this problem involves having a panel of children help in the selection of flavors. The development scientist must also face the unusual problem of finding flavors for products that will be acceptable to future customers. Taste preferences of people tend to change over a period of ten or more years. A product flavored with a fad or unusual flavor might, in time, lose customers because the flavor became less popular. More often, there is a gradual change in flavor preferences. Many established products with old-fashioned flavors receive continuing customer support in spite of their flavor.

Flavor involves taste sensation. It also involves the sensation of smell, touch, sight, and sound. There are four primary tastes: sweet, salty, sour, and bitter. The primary tastes are detected by special groups of cells called taste buds. These buds are located in the papillae — the little bumps — on the end of the tongue. Taste buds contain nerve endings which react with soluble flavors in the mouth. The impulses are transmitted by different nerves to the areas of the brain devoted to taste perception. The distribution of taste buds in the mouth and on the tongue changes as we get older. Infants and children have more taste buds in the mouth than do adults. This, in part, accounts for the different taste preferences of the little people. Sweetness and saltiness are detected by taste buds on the tip of the tongue while those on the sides of the tongue are most responsive to sourness; taste buds on the back of the tongue detect bitterness.

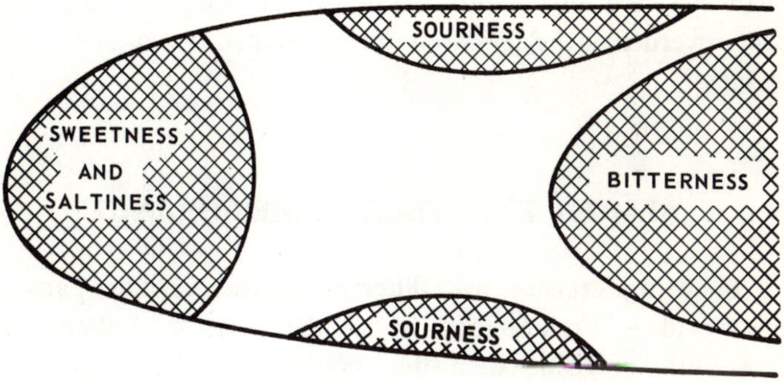

FIG. 6. Top view of tongue showing distribution of taste buds responsive to primary tastes.

The pathway for nerve transmissions from the buds is different. Sweetness and bitterness detectors each send messages to the brain by way of different nerves. The perceived taste sensation of flavored pharmaceutical products is an extremely complex phenomenon involving both intensity of taste and their duration.

Since flavor preferences are different for adults and for children, this point must be considered when formulating products for children. This requirement becomes especially important if the product is to be taken regularly. A good example would be a chewable vitamin tablet — the taste could very well decide whether or not children would willingly accept the "good" medicine day-after-day. This also poses a real problem for the development scientist: the flavor should be good enough so that the medicine will be taken willingly but not of such flavor that it would be mistaken for candy. Obviously, this problem must also be recognized by parents — medicines should *not* be identified as candy. To do so may lead children into thinking that all pleasantly flavored medicines are just candy. Many tragic cases of accidental drug overdosing in children have resulted from such carelessness.

ALMOST EVERYBODY LIKES ORANGE

Food preferences are different in the various parts of the world — French food is not the same as Italian food. It is not surprising then that people in different countries have their own ideas about what flavors are best. For example, the top three flavor preferences in pharmaceutical products in different countries around the world show some similarities and some interesting differences.

TOP THREE FLAVOR PREFERENCES FOR PHARMACEUTICAL PRODUCTS IN VARIOUS COUNTRIES

Germany	—	Orange, Peppermint, Anise
Norway	—	Anise, Chocolate, Licorice
Italy	—	Orange, Raspberry, Peppermint
Mexico	—	Orange, Lemon, Pineapple
Argentina	—	Orange, Lemon, Raspberry
Indonesia	—	Orange, Peppermint, Vanilla

The taste of drugs, and all other substances, can be broken down into an intensity factor and a duration factor.

The *how much* and *how long* concept of taste plays an important role in masking or covering up the taste of drugs in formulations. Most drugs are bitter — this seems to be a general rule, but, of course, there are important exceptions. The first thing a development scientist will do is determine intensity of the drug taste. This involves taste testing of progressive dilutions in order to determine at what concentration the taste of the drug is first detected. The more intense the taste of the drug, the lower the concentration that can be detected and the more difficult it will be to mask. For some intensely bitter drugs the average person can detect one part of drug in 10,000 parts of water. This value is known as the taste threshold. If the formulation requires one part

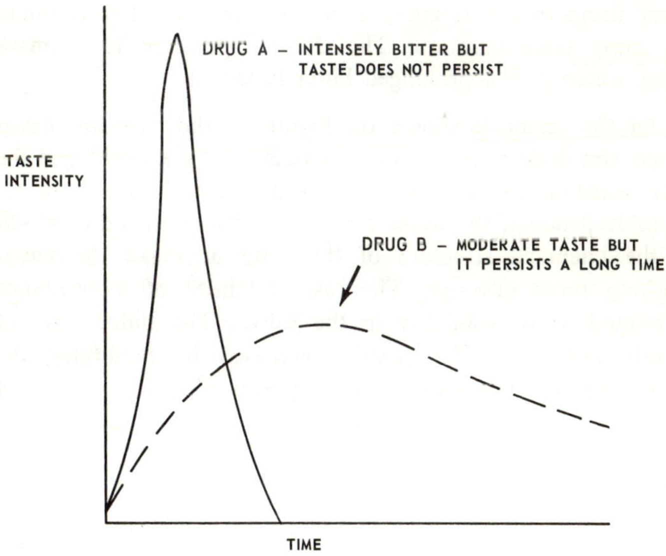

FIG. 7. Taste intensity of drugs as a function of time.

of the drug in 10 parts of water, the concentration will be 1000 over the taste threshold. Masking a flavor this intense presents a real problem!

After the taste threshold or limit of detection of a drug has been determined, it is then necessary to find out how long the taste persists. This may be done by tasting a standard solution of drug and rinsing out the mouth with water at various times. The object of the test is to find the time when the drug taste is no longer noticed. This difficult experiment must be done many times with different subjects using carefully controlled conditions to get reproducible values. Two different kinds of taste intensity profiles are shown in Figure 7.

Most of the popular flavoring agents are able to mask or cover drugs of the A group because these flavors have about the same taste duration. The difficult problem is to mask drugs which give a prolonged bitter taste.

In the example shown on Figure 8, the masking flavor covers the drug taste initially but tends to "wear off" and the bitter after-taste of the drug is then detected. To make an acceptable product, the development scientist must either modify the chemical structure of the drug or make the flavor masking more effective. The taste intensity of a substance is related to its solubility in the saliva. The bitter taste of certain drugs may be greatly decreased by modifying the drug to make it less soluble (see Fig. 9, p. 38).

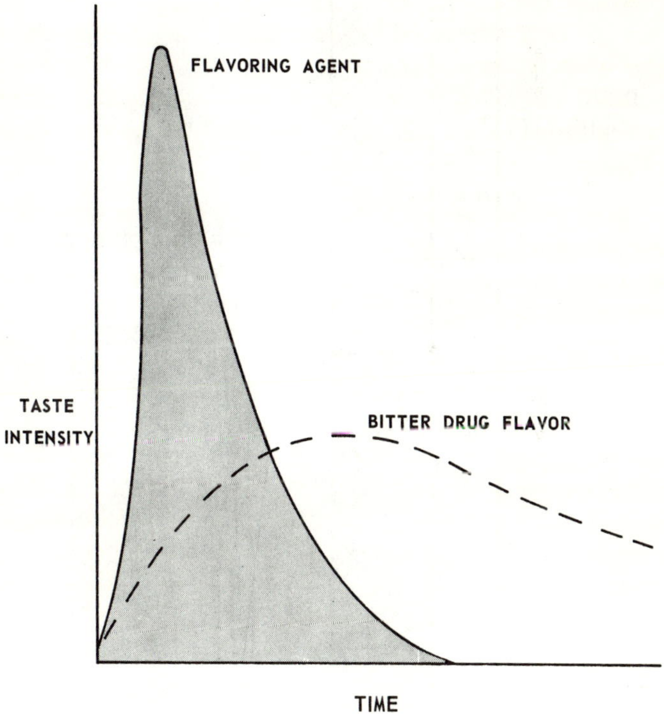

FIG 8. Taste intensity of a flavoring agent and a bitter drug as a function of time.

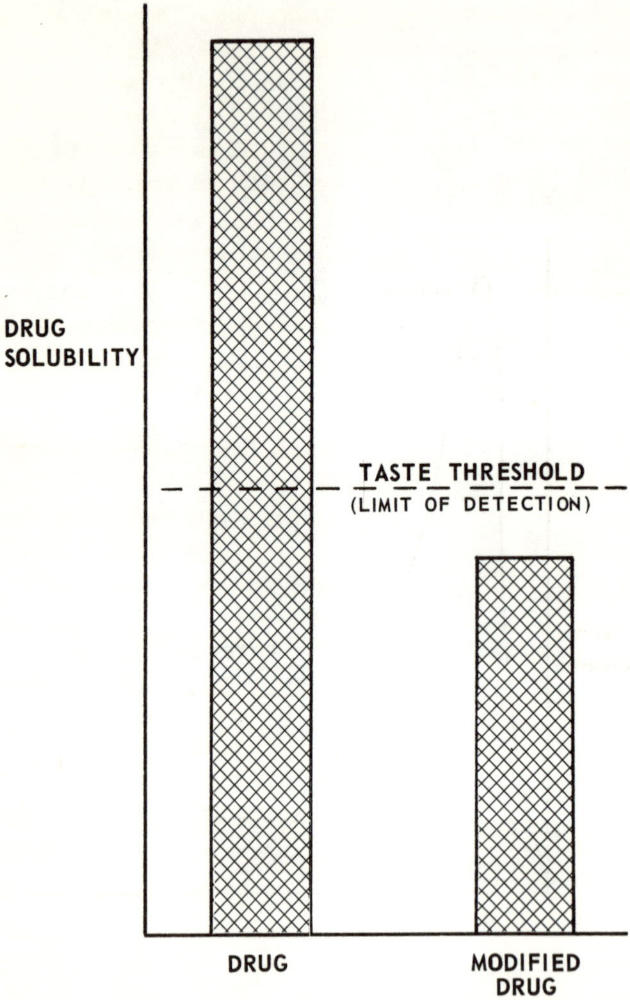

FIG. 9. Reducing the taste intensity of a drug by decreasing its solubility.

Chemical modification of the drug usually involves the formation of less soluble salts or derivatives. Another approach to taste masking involves making flavors persist longer by forming coated flavor granules that lodge on the surface of the tongue and then release the flavors gradually. This approach works best for certain kinds of solid dosage forms such as chewable tablets. For fluid products, the coating on the flavored granules tends to dissolve away before use. If the coating is made very thick to prevent this, the flavor is not released on the tongue. At best, it is a pretty tricky flavoring system. It does, however, illustrate the delicate balance of factors that takes place in each phase of product design.

Flavoring a product to appeal to the taste preferences of a lot of people leads, as we would suspect, to a lot of problems. The whole idea of flavoring is subjective. The person who tastes the flavored product may like, dislike, or be indifferent to it. His personal evaluation may not reflect how the majority of people would respond to the product. Often we do not know why we like a flavor — we just do.

A PANEL DECIDES

Flavoring a product might be done on the most subjective basis of all — by adjusting the flavor to suit the taste preference of the development scientist. The flavored product could then be given to another person for his taste evaluation. If this second person said that the taste was great, the development scientist would know that at least one person agreed with his choice of a flavor. He would not know how many others might like the flavor. In the same way, a rejection of the flavor by a single person doesn't really tell much — other than one for and one against. The development scientist improves his chances of finding an acceptable product flavor by sampling more people. He must be careful how he does this. For example, he can almost ensure taste panel approval by taking a sample around to his co-workers in the laboratory and saying, "try this new flavor — I'm sure you'll agree with me that it's great!" Chances are pretty good that they will agree with him if the question is asked this way. This might make him happy but would not provide much useful information about flavor acceptance by the consumer.

People on a taste panel and other consumer acceptance groups should reflect the preference of the people who will use the product. Even the preliminary laboratory test groups should have a balance between men and women and between typists and technicians. Samples of flavored products must be coded so that the taste panel members can't tell which is the boss's favorite. Careful development scientists have found that it is a good idea to check the results of the laboratory taste panel against taste panels in different parts of the country. Above all, it pays to check product acceptance in the age group who will use it: vitamin formulations designed for older persons should be taste-tested in the senior citizen group and pediatric products should be tested in children.

ALAS, THE COLOR IS GONE!

Pharmaceutical products are colored to make them more appealing, to provide protection, and to aid in their identification. Matching color with taste is one of the important ways to make a product appealing. Orange-flavored chewable vitamin tablets seem somehow to taste better when colored orange. Identification of tablets is greatly helped if tablets containing different drugs are colored differently. If all tablets were white, the chances of a patient making a mistake would be increased enormously. For people who must take several kinds of medicine, the color helps avoid mistakes. Of course, the label should be read carefully before taking any medication.

Selecting an appropriate color for a pharmaceutical product would seem, at first thought, to be relatively easy. Unfortunately, this is not so. Matching color with product flavor requires considerable skill. Proposed combinations must be checked in consumer acceptance panels. For fluid products, the panel might be asked to consider the pouring qualities and container appearance in addition to taste and color acceptance. The consumer panel would consider such factors as color, shape, and size for solid dosage forms.

Providing a different color for each different kind of tablet or fluid product is only part of the problem. The products should also be distinguishable from those made by other companies. If marketed internationally, the product must be distinguishable from similar products produced locally. For tablets — the most numerous of dosage forms — identification may be aided by printing the company's name on each tablet.

Color matching tablets and fluid products of the same drug is a special kind of challenge for the development scientist. The first problem encountered is that the same dye or colorant may not be available for use in the liquid and in the solid product. At the present time, there are only a limited number of coal tar dyes permitted by the U.S. Government's Food and Drug Administration for use in coloring liquids. Most tablets are colored by incorporating solid colorants into the formulation. These colorants are prepared by adsorbing approved dyes onto insoluble inorganic compounds.

THREE DIMENSIONS OF COLOR

We see the color of a liquid product as a combination of transmitted and reflected light. The color of a tablet is determined by reflected light as shown in Figure 10.

The colors may not appear to be identical even if the same dye is used in the fluid and in the tablet. Color matching by eye is a reasonably effective approach to the problem. Empirical or trial-and-error methods have certain disadvantages. They are unsatisfactory in the sense that no objective characterization of the color is available for future comparison. Quality of the product includes color — the best way to ensure quality is to express it in numbers.

Color is a three-dimensional concept involving *hue, lightness,* and *purity*. *Hue* is the attribute which distinguishes blue from red. *Lightness* of color on a gray scale from white to black differentiates light from dark objects. *Purity* is an intensity factor giving, say, the "blueness" of a blue. Values shown in Figure 11 range from 0 for perfect black to 10 for perfect white. On the circular line is given the full range of hues for red, yellow, green, and blue. The purity of any color is shown as a value from 0 to 10 on a line perpendicular to the lightness axis.

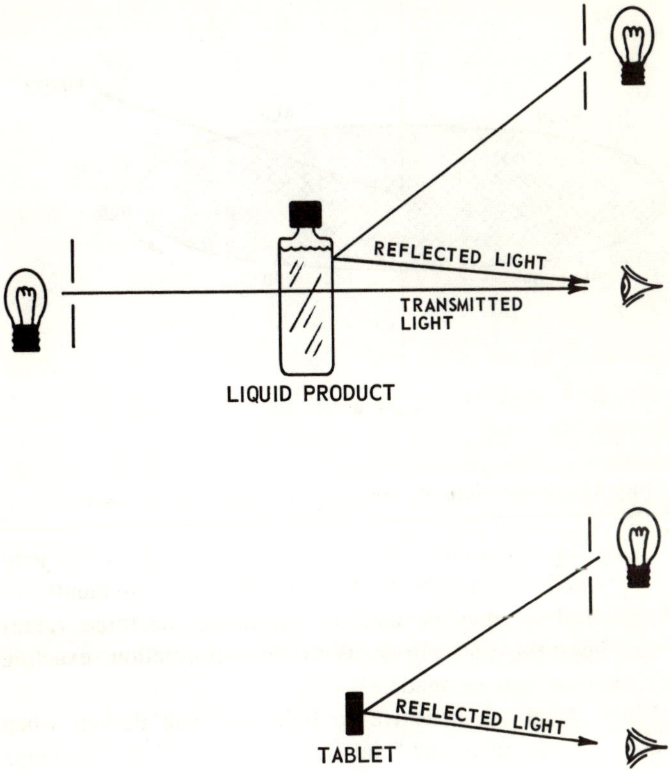

FIG. 10. Color perception of solid and fluid products.

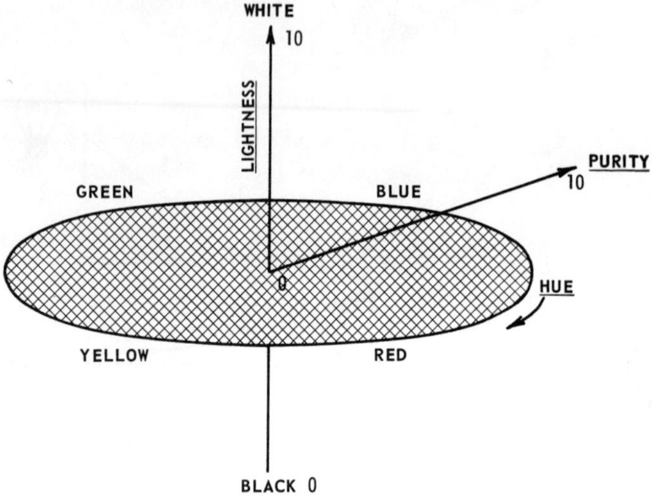

FIG. 11. Dimensions of color — the tristimulus concept.

Using this tristimulus concept, the color of an object may be expressed in numbers. Instrumental measurements of colored products may be used to determine the three values of hue, lightness, and purity. With this information, exacting color matches can be made.

Many drugs are sensitive to light and will darken when exposed to natural or artificial light. Even a slight darkening of white tablets will significantly decrease their eye-appeal. More important, any change in the appearance of the dosage form might be misinterpreted by the patient: he might think that the drug is no longer effective. Consumer confidence in a drug product is very important to the success of the product. Quality builds confidence — it must be an integral part of product design.

There are some obvious solutions to the problem of fading products like putting them in light-resistant containers. While effective, black bottles would certainly not be very appealing. Given a choice, the consumer always picks a product he can see! It is possible to change consumer preferences — but this generally requires a costly educational program. The waxed paper carton for milk has the advantage of being cheaper and disposable. Nonetheless, many people still prefer to buy milk in bottles because they can "see" what they are buying. Since seeing the product is considered important by the customer, opaque containers are used only as a last resort. Light-sensitive products may be packaged in amber colored glass containers. These permit the consumer to see the product and yet provide protection by filtering out light energies responsible for causing product breakdown. Beer is an example of a light-sensitive product usually sold in a colored bottle. The amber glass filters out the blue part of the spectrum responsible for deterioration.

With many pharmaceutical fluid products, it is possible to achieve light protection in clear glass almost equal to that of amber bottles by using appropriate coloring agents. The coloring agent must absorb harmful light rays without transferring this energy to the drug molecules. Light sensitivity of a fluid formulation, packaged in clear glass, may be tested by exposing samples to high intensity white light (Fig. 12).

Identification of pharmaceutical products is established only in part by the label and the container shape and size. What a product looks like, how it smells and tastes is of considerable importance. Regular users are sensitive to any change, however slight. Imagine the concern of a mother when she opens the familiar carton of vitamin drops and finds a bottle containing fluid that is yellow rather than the

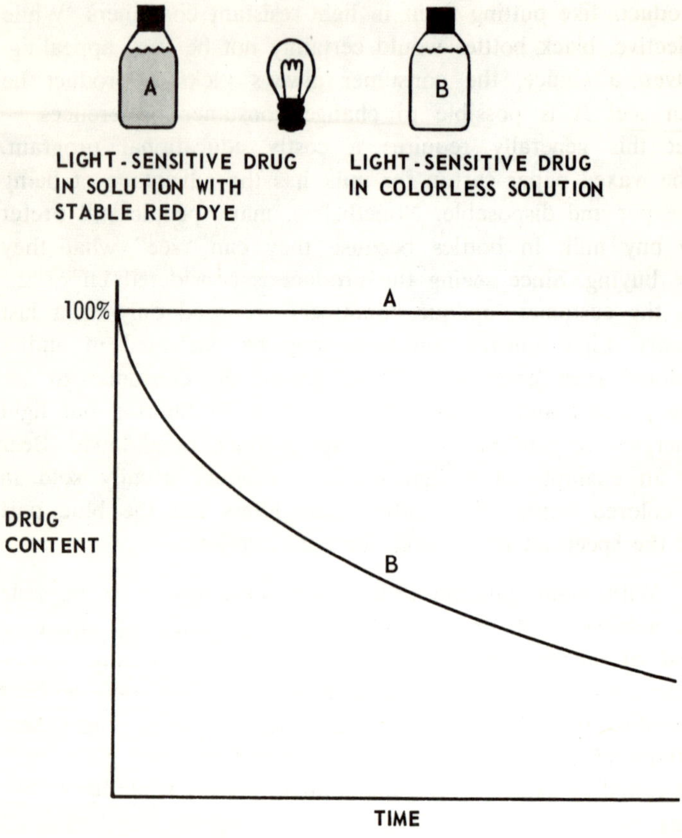

FIG. 12. Accelerated testing of light-sensitive fluid products.

expected bright orange color. Her first thought would be that the preparation had lost potency! It does little good to point out that color is not related to effectiveness. The problem of color loss is important simply because it causes consumer concern about the quality of the product. Consumer confidence is a vitally important factor for the success of any product. The consumer's concept of quality must always be considered in the design of pharmaceutical products.

We have pointed out that there are only a limited number of acceptable dyes available for use in coloring pharmaceutical products. Strict Government regulations apply to the use of these dyes in foods, beverages and drugs. The purity of the dye and the amount that may be used is carefully prescribed. The same requirements apply whether the dye is used internally in foods or in drugs. The amount of approved dyes consumed by the public in pharmaceutical products is exceedingly small compared to the quantities used in foods and beverages. Nonetheless, the same regulations apply to the red dye whether it is used in a beverage or in cough medicine.

Concern over the increasing use of various dyes in foods and beverages has prompted the Government to take a closer look at some of the approved dyes in this class. After extensive animal tests in which very large amounts of dyes were administered for long periods, certain dyes were delisted or discontinued from the Government approval list. All pharmaceutical products colored with such dyes had to be recolored with other approved dyes. The necessity of matching the established color of the product with acceptable new dyes posed a real challenge. Initial color matching is only one part of such a problem — not all dyes show the same light resistance. Substitute dyes must be checked for the trueness of color after storage under adverse conditions. Color of the product purchased by the consumer must match each and every time. If the color has faded, the quality may be questioned.

SQUEEZING TUBES AND POURING GOO

Design of a superior pharmaceutical product involves the balancing of formulation components and the selection of a suitable container. The formulation must be easily filled into the container during manufacture. Getting it out of the container is also important — the consumer is always concerned about getting what he pays for. He will not be satisfied with thick or viscous syrups that cannot be poured easily from the container. Equally annoying to the consumer is the problem of trying to open a tightly stuck cap or closure. A busy mother does not want to use pliers to open a bottle of cough syrup! Besides the annoyance factor, there is an important problem of economics — expensive materials that cannot be retrieved from the container make few friends for the product.

Fluidity of a product is a quality easily evaluated by the user. Indeed, the flow characteristics of the product may well determine consumer acceptance. Therefore, it should be no surprise that much effort has gone into measurement and control of flow properties of fluid and semi-solid dosage forms. There are many kinds of viscosity measurements. The simplest involves measuring the time for a fixed volume of fluid to flow through a certain sized opening. For example, the time for a funnel to drain empty might be 10 seconds when filled with water and 20 seconds when filled with a syrup. The *relative* viscosity of the syrup compared to water would be 20 seconds/10 seconds = 2.

The viscosity of fluid products may be increased greatly by additives. If we add two tablespoons of sugar to a cup of water, the resultant solution becomes more viscous or "thicker." It takes a lot of sugar to make the solution syrupy.

By contrast, the addition of two tablespoons of starch to hot water will make a thick paste. Most of the substances used to increase the viscosity of formulations are similar to starch — relatively small amounts are effective. Selection of the proper additive cannot be based solely on the viscosity effect produced in the formulation. Some of these viscosity-inducing substances interact with certain kinds of drugs to form poorly soluble salts or complexes. The development scientist must make certain that the viscosity-inducing agents in a formula do not bind or alter the effectiveness of the drug or other formulation components.

Accurate measurements of product properties such as viscosity are needed to ensure reproducible high quality in the making of fluid or semi-solid dosage forms. The quality introduced in the manufacturing step must be maintained over the expected life of the product. The development scientist must be certain that the viscosity of the product does not change significantly on storage. Imagine the problem caused by a product which, on standing, thickens to the point that the consumer cannot remove it from the container! He will be equally unhappy if the product becomes more fluid and squirts from the tube onto the floor with one squeeze. In either event, the user rarely buys the product a second time.

There is a dual requirement for ointment and cream formulations: getting them in and getting them out of the container. The "getting-in" problem usually occurs when a new ointment formulation is scaled-up for production equipment. Hand-filling a few tubes or jars with a very stiff ointment is no great problem so long as there is plenty of time. Filling thousands of containers may present formidable production difficulties. Ointment formulations must be designed to fill reproducibly at economical rates in standard production filling equipment. This requires careful measurement of the hardness or consistency of the formulation during development operations. Stiffness of ointments and other semi-solid products may be evaluated with a device known as a penetrometer. This is a simple apparatus which measures the penetration of a weighted cone into the material — the softer the material, the deeper the cone penetrates in a given period of time.

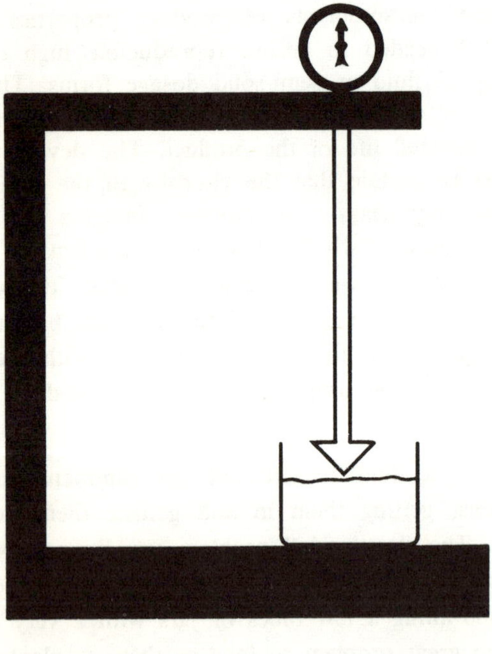

FIG. 13. The penetrometer — a device for testing ointment consistency.

The penetrometer is used to measure changes in the consistency of ointment bases at different temperatures. Typical results of such a study are shown below.

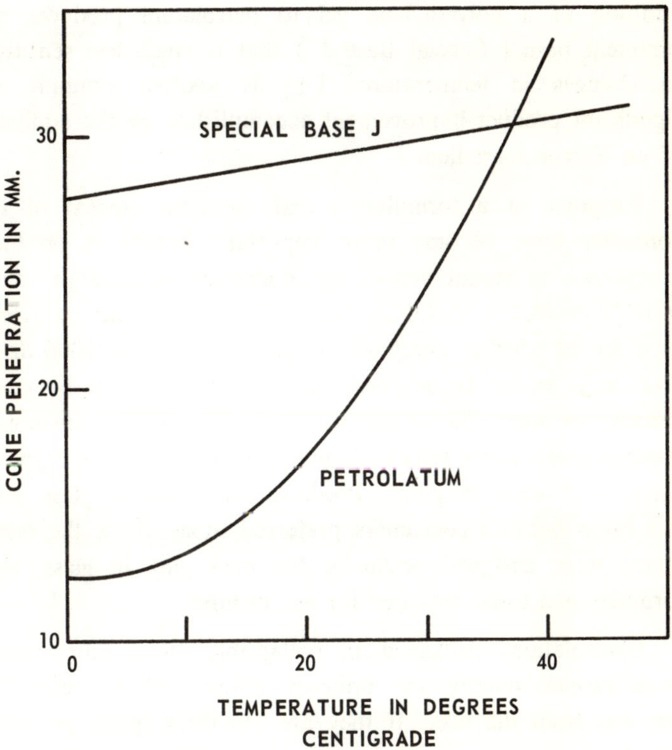

FIG. 14. Consistency of ointment bases as a function of temperature.

Petroleum jelly (petrolatum) ointment bases become much softer and more fluid at higher temperatures. The increased fluidity may permit suspended drug particles to settle to the bottom of the container. Separation of the active drug is an example of physical instability. Whenever dose uniformity is decreased, product quality is also decreased. The addition of a polyethylene gel to petrolatum produces an ointment base (Special Base J) that is much less sensitive to changes in temperature. This is another example of significant product improvement accomplished by the addition of an X-type ingredient.

Elegance of a formulation and consumer appeal of its container have become more important factors in product acceptance in recent years. The container or package must provide protection during storage so that the product performs as it should whether purchased 1 day, 100 days, or 1000 days after it is made. In addition, the container should be convenient to use. The consumer's ideas of what constitutes product convenience tend to change with time. Ointment packaging is a case in point. Products packaged in glass jars lost favor because consumers preferred tubes. Since the ointments were designed originally for packaging in glass, the formulas had to be modified for use in tubes.

Formulations packaged in collapsible metal tubes must have proper fluidity for uniform filling and for ease in removal from the tube. If they are too thick, great pressure will be needed to squeeze out some of the material; if too thin, the formulation will run out when the cap is taken off. Tube extrusion pressure for various experimental formulas is measured using the device shown in Figure 15.

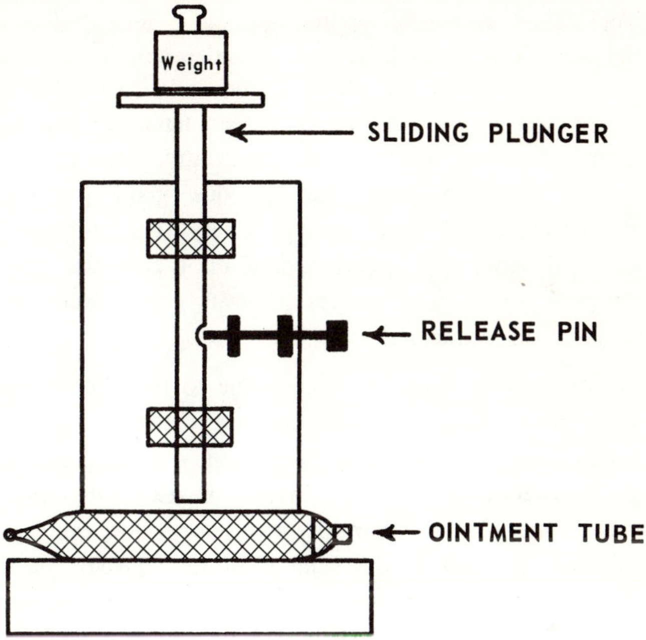

FIG. 15. Testing extrusion behavior of an ointment in a tube.

The tube is placed on the base and centered under the plunger. Weights are placed on the pan of the sliding plunger and then the release pin removed so that the weighted plunger pushes against the tube. The weight required to extrude 0.5 centimeter (about one-fifth inch) ribbon of ointment in 10 seconds is recorded. This value serves as a comparison standard for evaluating the flow property of different ointment bases from collapsible tubes.

THE CREAM "FEELS" GOOD

Topical or externally applied products must feel good on the skin. This is an important consideration for user acceptance. The purpose for which a product is designed determines the way it feels on the skin. Ointments are generally composed of a drug incorporated into a fatty, water-insoluble base like petroleum jelly; they provide good protection against moisture but tend to feel greasy. Creams have a similar consistency but are composed of a base that mixes readily with water. This makes removal much easier than is the case with ointments.

Creams may be thick or viscous due to the high content of active drug. They also must be easy to apply and have a smooth "feel" on the skin. Spreadability is an important design consideration for all topical or externally-applied products. One of the laboratory procedures for evaluating spreadability of such products involves putting some of the experimental formula on two glass slides and then squeezing them together like a sandwich. The excess is scraped off and the bottom held in place while the top slide is subjected to a pull of 80 grams. The time in seconds required to separate the slides is noted (see Fig. 16).

In addition to spreadability, such factors as ease of removal and non-staining of clothing are matters of real concern to the user. The sale of cosmetics and personal care products is determined largely by factors of customer convenience and acceptability. Consumer experience and satisfaction with the many excellent cosmetic products now available has raised the standards of acceptance for all products applied to the skin. Prescription products are no exception to this

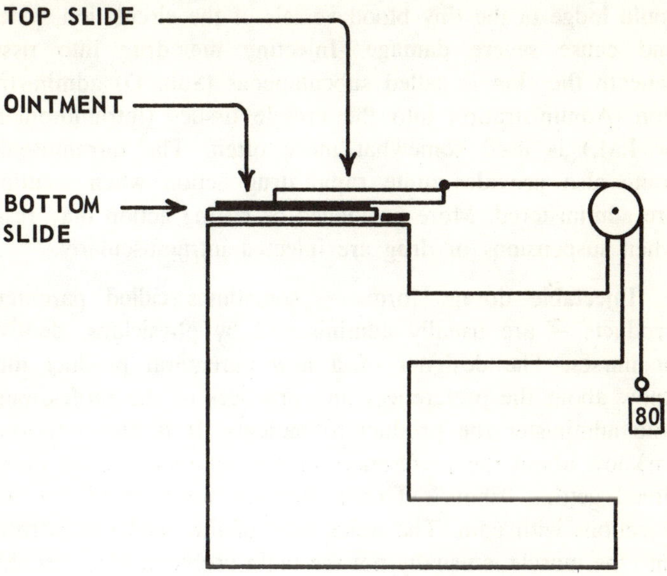

FIG. 16. Spreadability of an ointment — a laboratory test device.

rule — if the patient does not like the product, the doctor will soon prescribe another brand for the patient.

A SHOT IN THE ARM

Injectables are a special kind of dosage form meant to be administered by injecting the drug into the body by means of a needle and syringe. When the dose is injected directly into a vein, drug action is very rapid. Only completely clear solutions of drugs may be used for intravenous preparations. Any particles present in an intravenous (I.V.) product could lodge in the tiny blood vessels of the circulation system and cause severe damage. Injecting the drug into tissue beneath the skin is called subcutaneous (Sub. Q) administration. Administration into the muscle tissues (intramuscularly or I.M.) is used somewhat more often. The intramuscular route also provides quite rapid drug action when solutions are administered. More prolonged or lasting action may result when suspensions of drug are injected intramuscularly.

Injectable dosage forms — sometimes called parenteral products — are usually administered by physicians, dentists, or nurses. The designer of a new parenteral product must know about the preferences and practices of the professionals who administer the product to patients. It is also important to know about the preferences of the patients — most people dread getting "shots". This is because we tend to associate injections with pain. The quick hurt of the needle penetrating into the muscle is usually not the main problem. More troublesome is the persistent kind of burning pain associated with certain intramuscular injections. Long-lasting pain is generally due to the irritating action of the drug on muscle tissue. Proper formulation may greatly reduce the irritating action of many injectable drugs.

Injectable products *must* conform to one requirement: they must be sterile! In fact, these dosage forms are often called sterile products. Sterility or absolute freedom from microbial contamination may be achieved by heating the product to kill bacteria that are present or by filtering out the organisms using special filters. In addition to the sterility requirement, injectables should be completely free of fragments of killed bacteria and should not contain residues from microbial growth. The nitrogen-containing bacterial waste products are called pyrogens. These materials produce a mild fever if injected into a person, especially if administered intravenously. It is not enough to ensure that the injectable is sterile, it must also be free of pyrogens.

Putting the injectable product into a container is only one part of the development job. It is also necessary that the doctor or nurse be able to withdraw the full dose. Dose withdrawal is accomplished by putting the hollow hypodermic needle into the fluid and pulling back on the plunger of the syringe to suck up the fluid. The formulation must flow through hypodermic needles of the commonly-used diameters. If the product is made too thick or viscous, the effect may be like trying to suck up a thick malted milk through a narrow straw. Placing such products in disposable syringes is one way of avoiding the problem of withdrawing a dose from a vial. It is generally easier to push out a viscous fluid than it is to suck it up. Syringeability or ease of injection also must be tested. The disposable syringe must function well and deliver the full dose of drug under actual conditions of use.

The user of a product packaged in a multiple dose vial wants to be able to get out of the container the full number of doses stated on the label. This may be ensured by overfilling the container with a 10 per cent excess volume of the formulation. For thick or viscous suspensions, the additions of excess formulation may not solve the problem of draining time. Shaking the preparation to get good mixing before withdrawing a dose may have the effect of distributing the product all over the inner walls — this can make the dose withdrawal all but impossible. Coating the inner surface of the bottle with an extremely small amount of silicone improves draining characteristics.

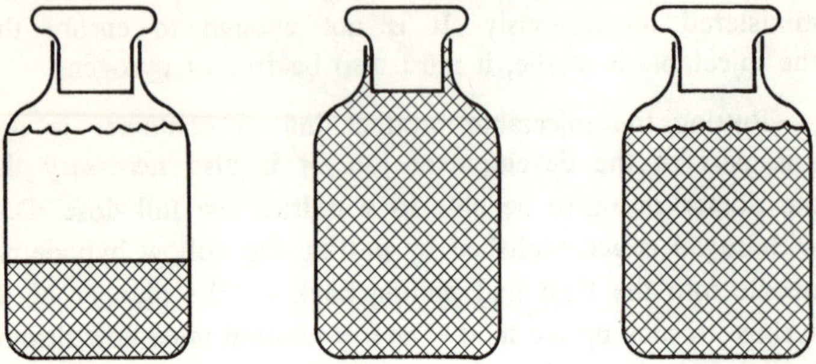

FIG. 17. Draining characteristics of ordinary and silicone coated vials.

Application of silicone coating to the surface of the bottle as a very thin film often provides dramatic improvements in wall draining. The silicones used for this purpose are effective and safe — another class of "inert" ingredients that might be properly called type X.

TABLETS FOR CHEWING AND SWALLOWING

Tablets are by far the most popular dosage form for administering drugs by mouth. They are especially useful because they provide an exact dose of drug that withstands storage for long periods of time with very little loss in potency. "Take a half tablet" is a familiar instruction from the physician. This may be done more easily if the tablets are scored.

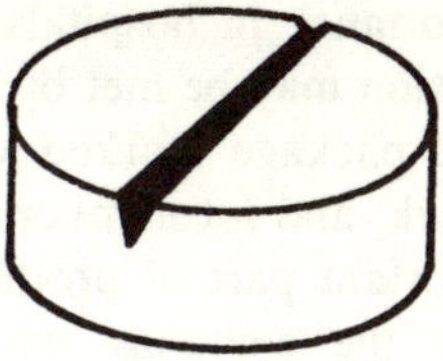

FIG. 18. Scored tablet — a way to give half the dose.

The tablet designer must balance this property of controlled breakability against the other important requirement that the tablets must hold together during packaging and storage. Sometimes the drug has a bitter taste or a bad odor. When this happens, the product development scientist may coat the tablet with a very thin film (no thicker than this page) to prevent the bitter taste from touching the tongue. Such film-coated tablets must be designed to provide taste protection without affecting the rapid release of the drug at the site of absorption.

Many people find it difficult to swallow large round tablets. Changing to an oval or capsule-shaped form may make the tablet seem easier to take. Altering the shape of a tablet may solve the patient acceptance problem. In solving one problem, a new one may be created: the new tablet shape may cause manufacturing difficulties which require a re-design of the formulation.

Tablets are made in special shapes and are colored, coated, and printed to provide easy identification. Reliable drug identification is important to the prescribing physician and to the pharmacist who dispenses the product. Most of all, identification helps the patient — especially the patient taking several kinds of drugs. Identifying different oral dosage forms may be of critical importance in hospitals and nursing homes. This need for identification may be met by placing each capsule or tablet in a separate package marked with the drug name, dose, company trademark, and lot number. Incidentally, this lot number is a most important part of product quality and identification — it permits the company who manufactured the product to check the identity of all ingredients used in the manufacture of that particular tablet.

Children — and many adults — have difficulty swallowing any kind of tablet, no matter how small. This is one of the major reasons for the popularity of the chewable tablet. For drugs that must be taken regularly, the chewable tablet has a special appeal. A chewable antacid tablet makes it possible for the ulcer patient to control the discomfort without having to take a glass of water to swallow the tablet. Preparations for controlling the symptom of coughs and colds are much more convenient in the form of chewable tablets.

Designing effective chewable tablets presents a special challenge for the development scientist. Processing factors must be balanced against the critical concern for patient acceptability. Above all, chewable tablets must be easy and pleasant to chew. Mouth feel and taste are particularly important. Addition of special sugars like mannitol and sorbitol help to give the soft, smooth, and non-sticky properties to such tablets. Chewable tablets must also stay chewable in storage. Proper formulation and careful package selection are necessary considerations in designing tablets that do not harden in storage. Chewing a rock-hard tablet may be a very unhappy experience if the teeth break before the tablet!

CHAPTER III

On The Shelf

PURITY

TODAY, full strength and purity of a drug product is taken for granted. This is as it should be! It is a matter of critical importance that the actual drug potency corresponds to the potency statement shown on the label. If the drug content of a product decreases significantly on storage, the patient may receive less than the prescribed amount of drug. This could have very serious consequences — the actual dose might be insufficient to effect a cure or to provide a proper level of treatment.

Maintaining drug potency in a dosage form presents an enormous challenge to the development scientist — many modern drugs are easily decomposed by the everyday condition of temperature, light, humidity, and even atmospheric oxygen. Stabilizing drug systems requires detailed information on how the drug loses potency and the rate at which this loss occurs. For example, an active drug molecule containing an ester linkage ($\text{-}\overset{\text{O}}{\overset{\|}{\text{c}}}\text{-o-}$) will hydrolyze or break down in water solutions.

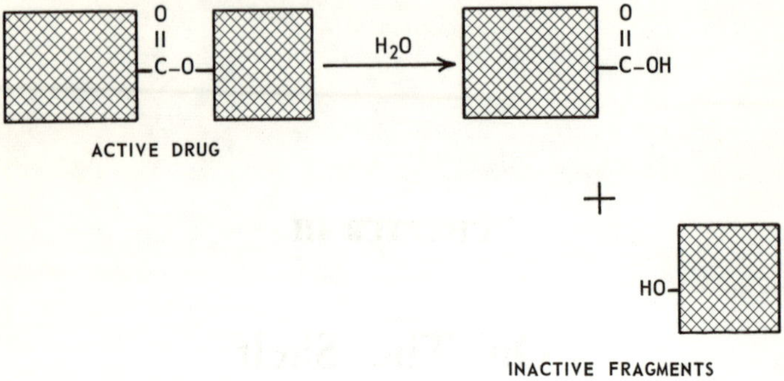

FIG. 19. Cleavage of an ester linkage — an example of drug decomposition.

The breakdown results in a loss in potency because the fragments or the cleaved drug molecule are not active. The amount of ester cleavage occuring in a unit of time increases in the presence of acids or bases. By measuring this rate of drug hydrolysis under different conditions of acidity or basicity, it is possible to construct the kind of curve diagrammed in Figure 20.

Information of this kind provides a starting point in the design of a proper formulation for the drug. The curve shows that for this particular drug, the greatest stability or least breakdown occurs at neutrality — numerically designated as pH 7. This sort of reaction rate profile permits the development scientist to calculate an amount of breakdown which would occur if the product were formulated in a somewhat more acidic fluid, say, at pH 5. Data of this kind are used in balancing stability against other formulation factors such as taste acceptance.

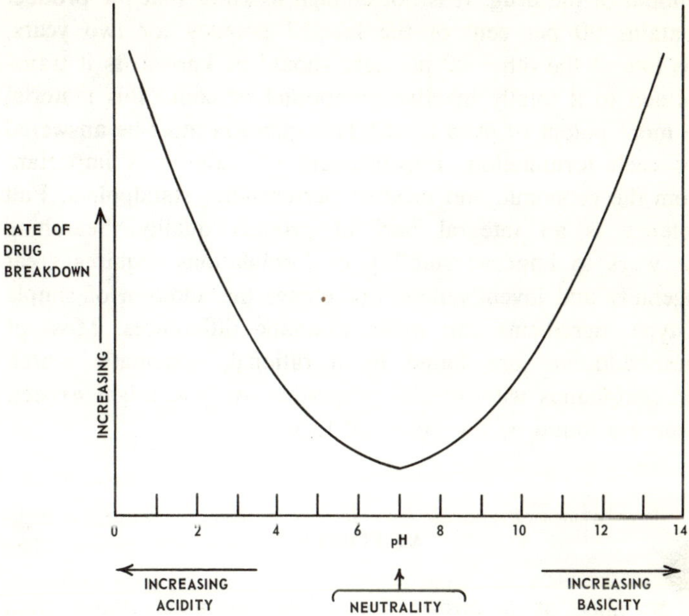

FIG. 20. A pH-rate profile — drug breakdown as a function of hydrogen ion concentration.

The breakdown of a drug in a dosage form generally occurs faster at higher temperatures. For this reason, many sensitive drug products must be stored in cool places or even refrigerated. The label on the product will indicate if any special storage conditions are required. Conditions for proper storage are determined by the development scientist before the product is marketed. He must also determine the expiration dating that should be put on the label of the product. An expiration date indicates the time that the product may be expected to contain not less than 90 per cent of the labeled amount of the drug. It is not enough to know that the product contains 90 per cent of the labeled potency for two years, the fate of the other 10 per cent should be known. Is it transformed to a totally inactive compound or could this material be more potent or even toxic? This question must be answered for each formulation. Improvement of stability is important from the economic and product performance standpoints. Full potency is an integral part of product quality. Searching for ways to improve stability of formulations requires great ingenuity and inventiveness. Sometimes the addition of simple X-type ingredients can make dramatic differences. Most of these additives are found by a rational, systematic search for compounds with special properties. As you might expect, some are found by the purest of luck.

ACTIVITY

Stability of a dosage form involves much more than simply making sure that all of the drug is present. The drug must be present in a form usable by the patient — it must provide the desired drug effect when taken. A tablet may exhibit excellent chemical stability in that no loss of drug occurs on long storage and yet not provide the expected full drug activity when taken. If a tablet does not disintegrate and permit its drug content to dissolve in the stomach or intestinal fluids, no drug absorption will take place. Without systemic absorption, the drug will not exert its intended effect. The end result is the same as if the drug in the tablet had deteriorated or lost potency.

Retention of original potency for long periods of time is one of the characteristics of an ideal dosage form. Longer shelf life for a product can easily be translated into higher quality: the product is at full potency and ready for use when needed. Products with a longer shelf life generally provide a better economic picture in that fewer lots of material need to be manufactured to ensure that full potency products are always available to the consumers. This means lower product prices and consumer savings.

STOCKPILES AND DOCTORS' BAGS

Stockpiling of essential drugs for national emergencies has, in the past decade, provided a great stimulus for the design of unusually stable drug products. Drugs in this category must be on hand in large quantities since the capacity to produce additional supplies might be seriously hampered by an emergency. Considerable expense would be involved in the initial stockpiling of large quantities of an essential drug product. If this stock retained potency for only one year, the cost to maintain an inventory over a ten-year period would be ten times the original stock cost. Increasing the stability or shelf life of such a product to five or even ten years would result in enormous savings. This is the kind of problem that makes development of dosage forms a real challenge. Finding and testing simple additives that will extend the shelf life of drug products can be equally as important as finding new drugs.

Many dosage forms must be relied upon to retain their potency under rather adverse conditions. Knowing what kind of conditions a product may encounter is important in designing tests to predict product shelf life. When thinking of extremes of temperature and humidity, the first thoughts that come to mind are those of tropical countries, ocean voyages, and unheated warehouses in the northern climates. Shipment and storage of drug products in exotic and faraway locations places stringent requirements on the stability of the products. This, of course, is a well-recognized problem. Not so obvious are the adverse conditions encountered in storage of drug products in seemingly safe places. The family "medicine" cabinet may subject drug products to humidities as high as those found in rain forests. The drugs normally carried by the physician in his bag are carefully selected emergency-type drugs which must be absolutely reliable and ready for instant use. Since the bag is normally carried in the trunk of the physician's auto, the drugs are exposed to the extreme heat of summer and the cold of winter. Exposure of drug products to similar cycling temperatures of cold and hot must be carried out in the laboratory during the testing of the experimental formulations. Every effort must be made to make certain that deterioration does not occur under actual storage conditions.

Knowing about the ways that drug products are stored in actual practice helps a pharmaceutical scientist to design valid product tests. Evaluation of the product involves both formula and container. The laboratory test should give reliable information about the stability of an experimental formulation in less time than it would take by actual storage of the proposed product at room temperature. Accelerated testing involves the measurement of chemical and physical properties of a formulation subjected to temperatures higher than normal. Measurement is the key word! To know something about a system, it is necessary to measure it — knowledge of physical systems that cannot be expressed in numbers is neither complete nor satisfying to a scientist.

EARLY WARNING SYSTEM

Making time go faster – can this be done? No, not really. We are able to speed up certain degradative processes by changing conditions. By increasing the storage temperature we are able to find out how much drug deterioration may be expected to occur in a dosage form when it is exposed to normal temperatures. Comparing the drug stability of experimental formulations at room temperature is a slow operation.

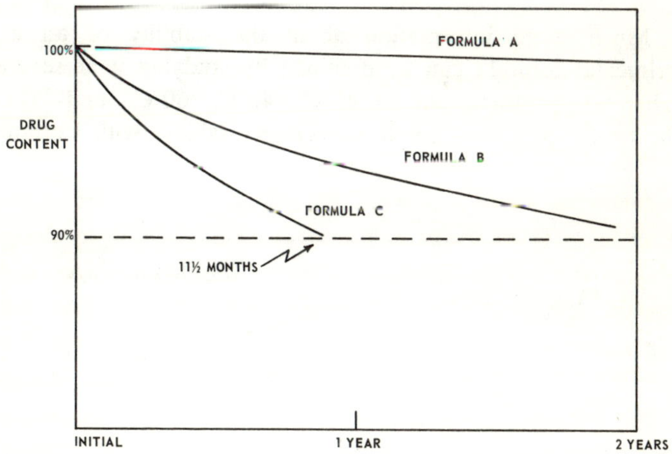

FIG. 21. Stability of experimental drug formulations at room temperature (25°C).

Waiting for two years would be a sure way of knowing which formula to pick but this would result in unnecessary delay. It is possible, though, to study the stability of the same formulas at several higher temperatures and make a good prediction of their stability at room temperature.

An "early warning" of the stability of a drug product can be obtained in about a month but the prediction is considerably improved if the study is carried out for two months. Application of the principles of chemical kinetics to predict drug stability will be illustrated for the case of Formula C. Actual shelf life of this experimental product was about 11 1/2 months at room temperature. This, of course, is the most reliable information but it takes almost a year to get it. Worse yet, the shelf life would not be satisfactory and, if no other formulas were made, the project would be almost one year behind schedule.

Much more information about the stability of an experimental formula can be obtained by studying it at several higher temperatures, say at 42°C., 46°C., 60°C., and 70°C. The results of a two-month accelerated stability with Formula

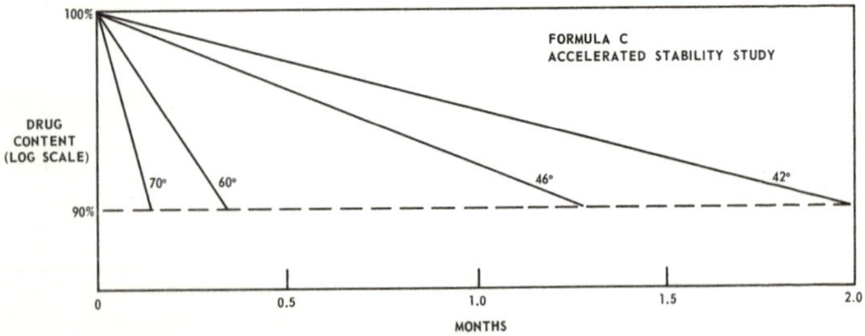

FIG. 22. Stability of an experimental drug formulation at different temperatures — an accelerated test method.

C are shown in Figure 22. Note that drug content decreased at a faster rate at the higher temperatures.

The data shown above are used to make a new graph from which the actual prediction is then made. In order to do this, the values must be replotted in such a way that a linear or straight line relationship is obtained. We will not go into the theoretical details of this. The following brief mathematical romp only serves to show how numbers are rearranged by scientists to provide more information about the stability of drug systems. First of all, the time in months for the formula to decline to 90 per cent of its initial drug activity at various temperatures must be determined. This time value is then expressed as reciprocals — a form proportional to the rate constant for the reaction:

Temperature (Degrees Centigrade)	Time in Months for Drug Content to Fall to 90% (*t*-90%)	Reciprocal of *t* 90%
42°	2 months	$\frac{1}{2.00 \text{ mo.}} = 0.5 \text{ mo.}^{-1}$
46°	1.3	$\frac{1}{1.30 \text{ mo.}} = 0.77 \text{ mo.}^{-1}$
60°	0.35	$\frac{1}{0.35 \text{ mo.}} = 2.85 \text{ mo.}^{-1}$
70°	0.14	$\frac{1}{0.14 \text{ mo.}} = 7.15 \text{ mo.}^{-1}$

Next, the temperatures are converted to absolute or Kelvin scale by adding 273° to the Centigrade temperatures; the reciprocal of the absolute temperature is then determined.

Temperature (Degrees Centigrade)	Absolute Temperature (Degrees Kelvin)	Reciprocal of Absolute Temperature
42°	+ 273 = 315°K	$\frac{1}{315} = 0.00317$
46°	+ 273 = 319°K	$\frac{1}{319} = 0.00313$
60°	+ 273 = 333°K	$\frac{1}{333} = 0.00300$
70°	+ 273 = 343°K	$\frac{1}{343} = 0.00291$

Finally, the reciprocals of the times for drug content to fall to 90 per cent (1/t-90 per cent) are plotted on the *Y* axis of a log scale graph against the reciprocal of absolute temperature on the *X* axis. This is shown in Figure 23.

The intersect of the extrapolated (dashed) line to room temperature occurs at a value of (1/*t*-90 per cent) equal to 0.09 months^{-1}. This corresponds to a predicted shelf life of 11.1 months at room temperature (25°C.):

$$\frac{1}{t\ 90\%} = 0.09 \text{ months}^{-1}$$

$$t\ 90\% = \frac{1}{0.09 \text{ months}^{-1}} = 11.1 \text{ months}$$

The predicted value shows good agreement with the actual value of 11.5 months and has the advantage of being obtained in two months.

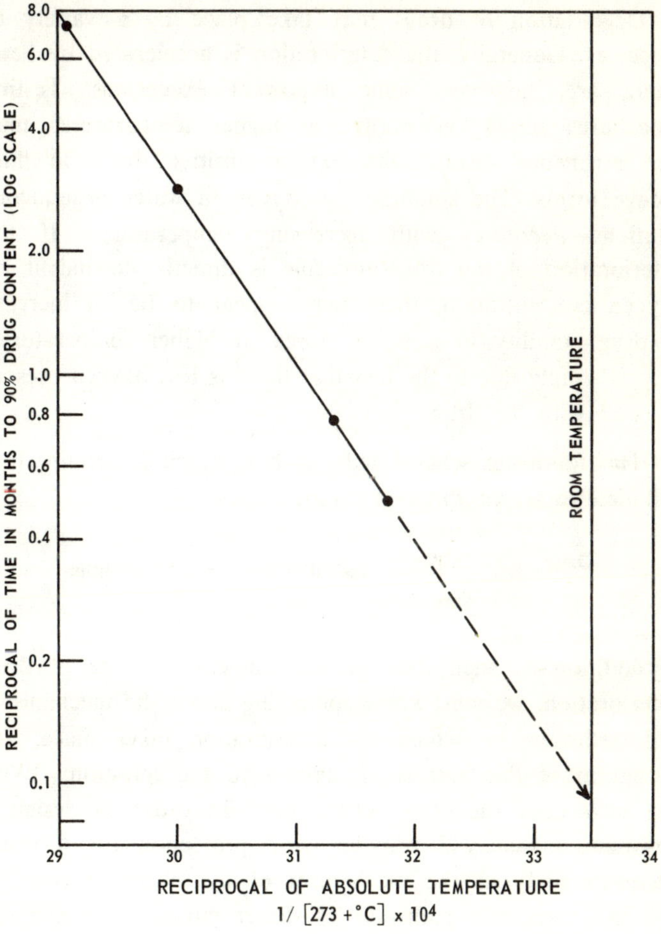

FIG. 23. Predicting room temperature stability of a drug formulation from high temperature data — an Arrhenius plot.

MECHANISMS AND PATHWAYS

Degradation of drugs may take place by a variety of processes. Generally, the deterioration is accelerated by heat. There are, however, some important exceptions. Testing procedures based on storage at higher temperatures may give erroneous results with oxygen-sensitive drugs in fluid dosage forms. The solubility of oxygen in water or aqueous solutions *decreases* with increasing temperatures. If the deterioration of the drug molecule is directly dependent on oxygen concentration, there may appear to be an increase in drug stability in samples stored at higher temperatures. This is simply due to the fact that there is less oxygen present to react with the drug.

The following scheme tells us how much a certain drug will deteriorate at different temperatures:

$$\text{Drug} \xrightarrow{25°\text{C.}} 10\% \text{ Loss in } 11.5 \text{ months}$$

$$\xrightarrow{70°\text{C.}} 10\% \text{ Loss in } 4.2 \text{ days}$$

In addition to such data on the velocity or rate of drug deterioration, we must know something about the mechanisms and pathways by which the deterioration takes place. Information of this sort is an answer to the question: "Why and how does the drug deteriorate?" In order to design a formulation that will provide good protection for a drug, we must find out the mechanism of the chemical reaction and the respective pathways of deterioration. For example, at a given temperature, the drug may decompose or lose potency by three competing reactions:

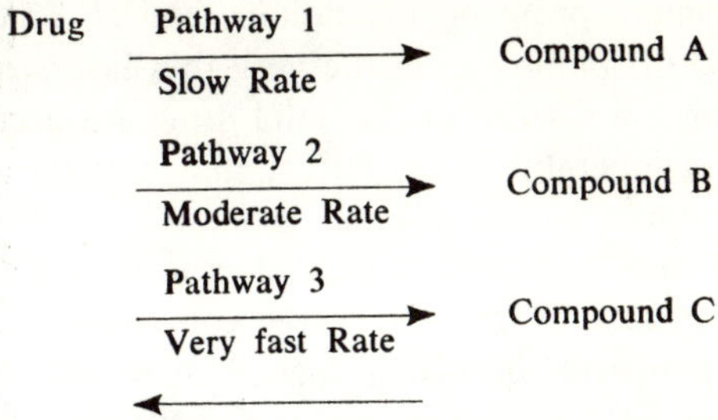

While the reaction along Pathway 3 occurs at a very fast rate, this does not necessarily mean that this is the principal route of degradation. In fact, it may result in no significant loss of activity. Note that the reaction is reversible — compound C reverts to original active drug. If Pathway 2 were shown to be an oxidative reaction, it might be possible to greatly reduce the rate of drug loss by adding a suitable antioxidant or by improving the containers for the formulation. Knowing about the pathways of loss is an essential part of devising counter measures. We must also know how much loss occurs by the respective pathways — a maximum effort to control the slow loss by Pathway 1 would have little effect on overall drug stability.

AIR, AIR — EVERYWHERE

When a drug is susceptible to breakdown in the presence of oxygen, the design of a stable dosage form presents formidable problems. Air contains about 20 per cent oxygen and it is everywhere! Administering an oxygen-sensitive drug in a solid dosage form avoids many — but not all — degradation problems. Keeping moisture away from the drug then becomes the primary problem. Oxidations, and all other reactions, take place in solution — in the very thin layers of moisture adsorbed on the surface of the solid drug. An accelerated test using high temperature, say 60°C., may dry the powder to such an extent that the normal oxidative reaction does not occur. This may be due to a lack of moisture on the surface of drug crystals or to the decreased oxygen solubility at the higher temperature. Using higher than normal pressures of oxygen in an accelerated test may give a better indication of drug stability.

The scale-up of formulations containing oxygen-sensitive drugs is extremely difficult. Formulations made in large production-type equipment often do not exhibit the same stability as when made in small quantities using laboratory-scale equipment. This discrepancy may be due to a variety of reasons. Slight differences in stirring times or heating rates may greatly affect the product quality. For this reason, it is especially important to check the stability prediction for laboratory-sized quantities against full production-sized lots.

The passage of atmospheric oxygen through containers made of certain types of plastics occurs surprisingly fast. The storage time of oxygen-sensitive drugs in such containers may be less than the 24-month minimum requirement. Placing solutions of oxygen-sensitive drugs into tightly capped glass bottles will reduce drug decomposition — until the bottle is opened. Each time the bottle is opened, the oxygen in the air headspace above the solution is renewed. The same problem occurs with multiple dose parenteral products because an equal volume of air must be injected into the vial to permit withdrawal of the dose.

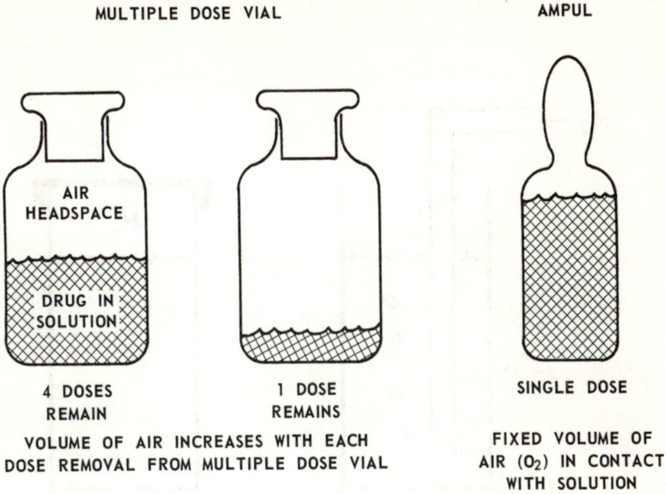

FIG. 24. Air contact with injectable products.

Ampuls or sealed glass vials contain a single dose of drugs – the solution is in contact with a limited amount of air until ready for use. To remove the dose of drug, the ampul must be broken open by snapping the thin glass neck. Ampuls provide outstanding protection of contents but they are not especially convenient to use. This illustrates again the ever-present problem of balancing factors.

Bubbling an inert gas like nitrogen through a drug solution is an effective way of decreasing the amount of oxygen present in the system. The nitrogen displaces the oxygen from solution. If the container holding the drug solution is quickly sealed after nitrogen is bubbled through it, there will be very little oxygen in the solution or in the headspace.

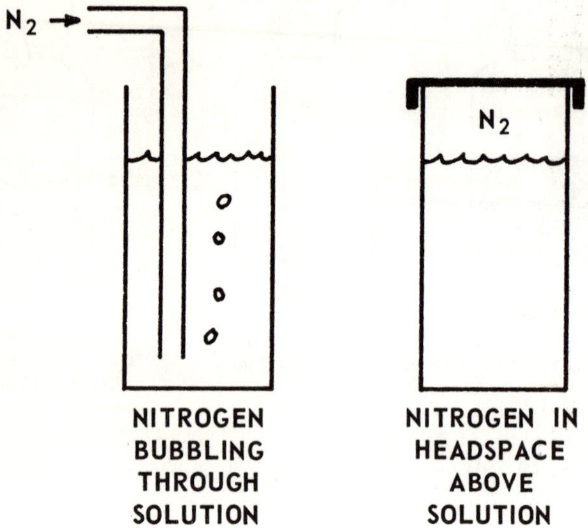

FIG. 25. Oxygen removal from drug solutions by displacement with an inert gas.

When the container is opened, this protection against oxygen is lost in a matter of minutes. The rapid diffusion of oxygen back into the drug solution can be demonstrated in a very dramatic fashion by using a compound that changes to a blue color in the presence of oxygen. When sealed containers are carefully opened, it will be seen that the surface of the liquid quickly turns blue. The speed with which oxygen penetrates or diffuses into the unstirred solution may be measured by noting the depth of the colored band.

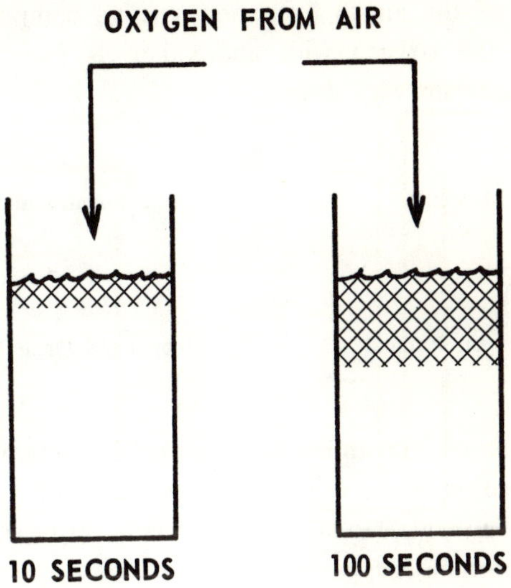

FIG. 26. Diffusion of oxygen into drug solution.

OXYGEN SCAVENGERS

Oxidation usually takes place by a chain reaction. One reactive oxygen radical reacts with one drug molecule to form a reactive compound which, in turn, reacts with another drug molecule. The process is repeated over and over again resulting in a rapid breakdown of drug:

Reactive Oxygen Radical* + Drug Molecule ⟶ Reactive Compound*
Reactive Compound* + Drug Molecule ⟶ Reactive Compound* + Reactive Compound*

Antioxidants are substances added to formulations to protect the drug from oxidation. Generally antioxidants react with the oxygen of the air to form non-reactive compounds. The reaction of the oxygen with antioxidant is faster than the reaction of oxygen with drug:

[Antioxidant Molecule + Drug Molecule + Reactive Oxygen Radical*] → Inactive Antioxidant Molecule + Unchanged Drug Molecule

The presence of the antioxidant in the formula may make the difference between a marginal product and one having full potency and high quality. Antioxidants represent another class of important X-type ingredients.

Oxidation reactions are often accelerated by the presence of trace amounts of such metal ions as copper or iron in the system. Certain compounds are capable of binding these metal ions in such a way that the ions are no longer capable of speeding up oxidative reactions. Adding such binding or sequestering agents to oxygen-sensitive formulations may greatly increase the shelf-life of the product. Selecting the proper sequestering agent requires the same systematic evaluation that is used for all formulation components; that is, the additive must perform its intended function without adversely affecting the performance of the active drug component or the other formulation ingredients. As with all other additives, it must not affect the safety and reliability of the product.

LIGHTS OUT

Sensitivity to light is a common degradative pathway for many drug molecules. Liquid dosage forms for such drugs normally are colored to absorb those wave lengths of light responsible for the drug's destruction. To be fully effective, the dyes used for this purpose should absorb the light energy without transferring it to the drug molecules. Solid dosage forms like tablets are provided with colored opaque coatings for the same reason. The container also plays a big role in protecting the product from light — this is the reason many kinds of drug products are packaged in amber-colored glass bottles. Accelerated testing of light-sensitive drugs in experimental formulations involves exposing the product, in different containers, to special experimental light conditions. High intensity white light corresponding to the spectrum of natural sunlight is used in these accelerated light tests.

CHECKING PREDICTIONS

No matter what kind of accelerated stability test is used, it must be validated against actual storage conditions. Checking predictions is done by regular analysis or assay of the drug in experimental formulas stored at room temperature. Simulating actual use conditions occasionally reveals some failings of the experimental formula that were not readily apparent by the standard accelerated stability test. An example of this would be a liquid product designed to be given in teaspoon doses: flavor losses may be very pronounced if the container is opened three times every day until used up. The normal test procedure would miss important information if only full containers were used in the tests for flavor and odor quality. This technique of repeated sampling from the same container often reveals unexpected problems like sticking caps on bottles containing syrups.

CAGES FOR MOLECULES

The molecular structure of certain substances resembles a cage. If the dimensions of the molecular cage are just right, a drug molecule may fit inside of the cage. These compounds are unique in that they are not formed by chemical reaction. The primary requirement for their formation is a proper match between the dimensions of the guest molecule and the host molecule.

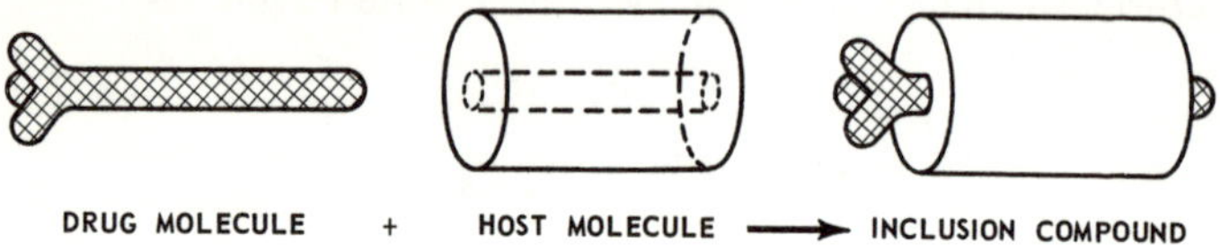

FIG. 27. Protected inclusion compound formed by interaction of a drug molecule with a host molecule of appropriate dimensions.

Inclusion compounds are sometimes called clathrate (meaning cage-like) compounds because the structure of the host molecule resembles a cage. The usefulness of clathrate compounds for protecting sensitive drugs has been demonstrated by pharmaceutical scientists. Reports of their investigations have appeared in *The Journal of Pharmaceutical Sciences.* Perhaps the most extraordinary aspect of the clathrate or inclusion compounds is that many provide protection for the guest molecule even in solution. Some host molecules are in the form of a flexible helix — much like a coiled telephone cord. Drug molecules of proper dimensions may fit into this helix in the same way a pencil will fit inside the coiled telephone cord.

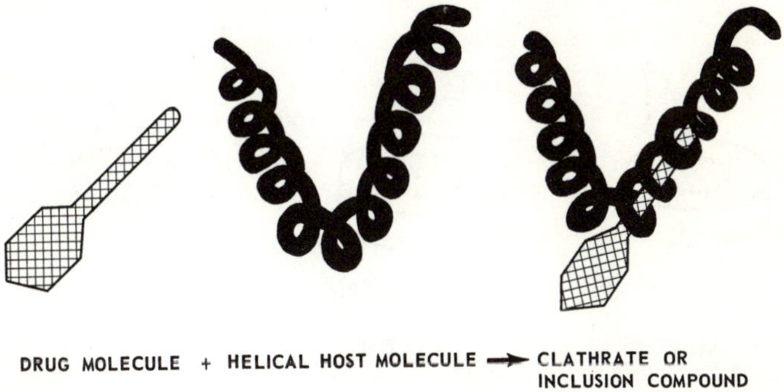

FIG. 28. Clathrate compound formed by the accommodation of a helical host polymer to a drug molecule.

The bulky size of the inclusion compound provides protection by preventing the reactive agent (oxygen, other molecules or ions) from coming into close contact with the drug molecule.

Certain kinds of organic compounds are capable of including molecular gases such as carbon dioxide within their cage-like structure. The inclusion of gases as within the cage structure of the host molecule provides a unique method for storing gases at normal temperatures and pressure in a solid form. The gas may be released by heating the compound to disrupt the clathrate structure or by dissolving the compound in a suitable solvent. The concentration of a gas stored in such solid clathrates would exert a pressure of 90 atmospheres if stored in a container of similar volume.

Cyclodextrins are a unique kind of inclusion host compound. They are made up of six, seven, or eight glucose units formed together in a shape like a doughnut. The different cyclodextrins are known respectively as ALPHA, BETA, AND GAMMA each of which have different diameter holes.

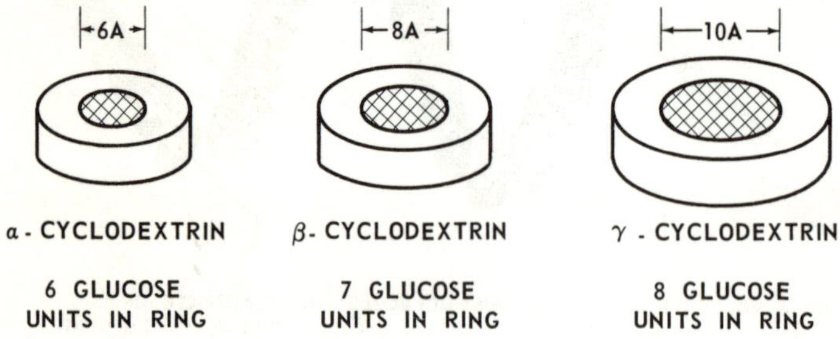

FIG. 29. Doughnut-shaped cyclodextrin host molecules capable of forming inclusion compounds with certain drugs in solution.

Cyclodextrins form inclusion compounds with guest molecules of appropriate size — the guest molecule fits inside the doughnut hole. For example, ALPHA-cyclodextrin has a doughnut hole about 6 Angstroms in diameter; it forms inclusion compounds with benzene derivatives having small substituent groups. The GAMMA form of cyclodextrin with its larger cavity of 10 Angstroms forms adducts or inclusion compounds only with larger organic molecules that give a good fit, inside the doughnut hole.

The simple organic molecule urea ($H_2N\ C\ O\ NH_2$) forms a special canal type clathrate in the presence of certain guest molecules. The interconnected urea molecules are arranged like wax in a honeycomb.

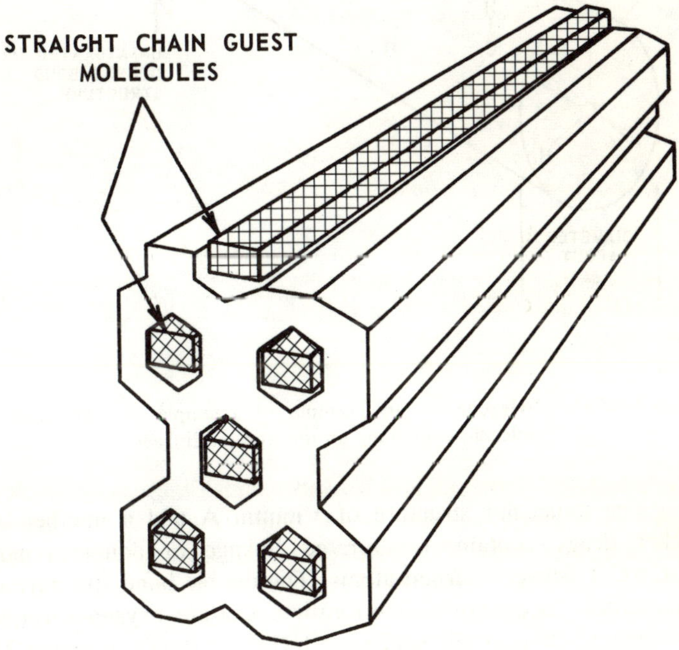

FIG. 30. Stabilized straight chain molecules contained in a canal-type urea clathrate.

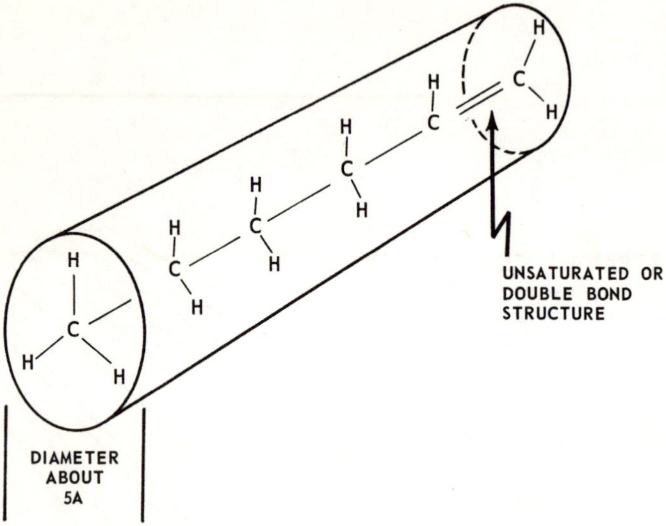

FIG. 31. 1-Hexene — an example of a simple straight chain molecule containing an unsaturated linkage.

The molecular structure of Vitamin A and a number of other drugs contain unsaturated linkage or double bonds (-C=C-) between carbon atoms. The double bond structure is susceptible to oxidative deterioration. Certain oxygen-sensitive compounds structurally similar to 1-Hexene shown in Figure 31 may be protected against decomposition by forming channel clathrates. The most important requirement is that of molecular dimension — the guest molecule must fit into the channel.

The local anesthetic drug, benzocaine, undergoes gradual cleavage or hydrolysis in aqueous solutions.

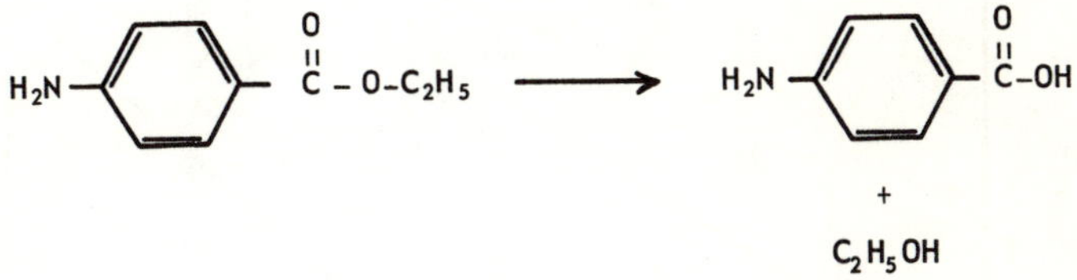

FIG. 32. Breakdown of the drug benzocaine in water — a hydrolytic reaction.

This hydrolytic breakdown may result in a significant loss of drug potency over a period of time. Drug decomposition by this mechanism or pathway may be prevented by adding caffeine to the solution to form a caffeine-benzocaine complex. Detection of such complexes in solution is achieved by measuring the solubility of the drug in the presence of the complexing agent.

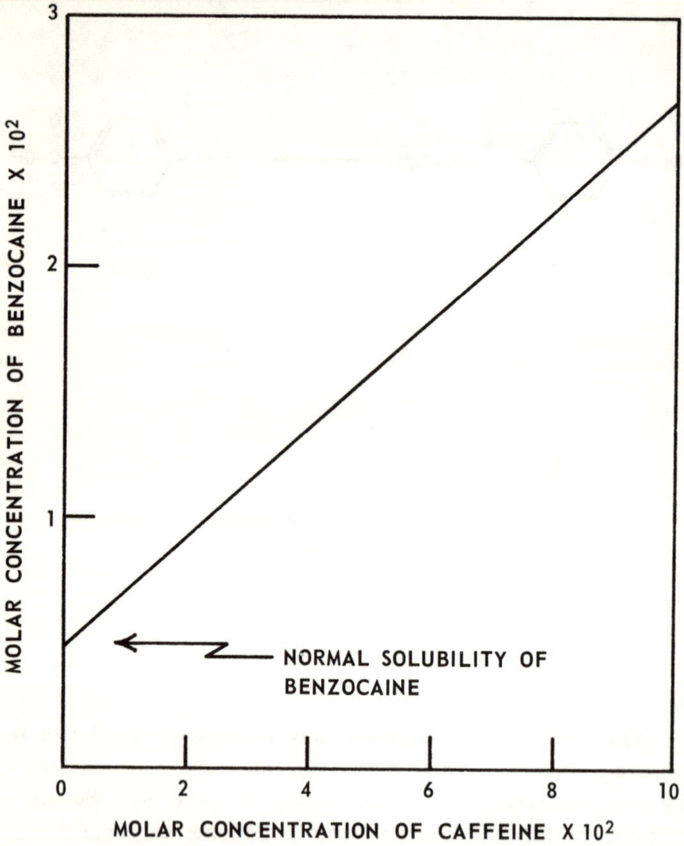

FIG. 33. Detecting the soluble complex benzocaine-caffeine by measuring benzocaine solubility in the presence of caffeine.

The solubility increase of benzocaine is found to be directly dependent on the concentration of caffeine — the complex contains one molecule of benzocaine and one of caffeine. The complex does not undergo hydrolysis to any significant extent. Only the free or uncombined benzocaine breaks down. The influence of caffeine on the rate of hydrolysis of benzocaine is shown below.

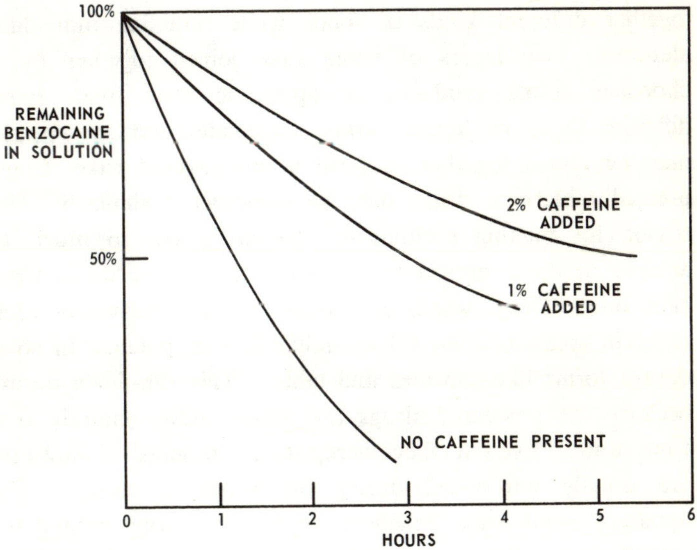

FIG. 34. Retarding benzocaine breakdown by adding caffeine to form a stable complex.

At a concentration of only 2 per cent added caffeine in the system, the hydrolytic rate is reduced to about one-fifth that of the unprotected solution. Caffeine is found in many cola beverages, in coffee, and in tea. It fulfills one of the important requirements of an ideal X-type ingredient in that it has a low order of toxicity and has been widely used by humans without serious effects.

LAYER CAKES

Layered cakes are a most pleasing way of putting together different kinds of foods while retaining individual identities. Two layers of white cake joined together by a chocolate filling produces an appealing taste treat. Even different kinds of layers (white, chocolate, and strawberry) may be joined together to form a multilayered cake. Compressed tablets of drugs may be constructed similarly. The reason for making multilayered tablets is not so much to achieve aesthetic appeal but to separate reactive drugs from each other. Drugs which deteriorate in the presence of each other in solution often show similar loss of potency in solid dosage forms like capsules and tablets. This run-down occurs because the powdered drugs are almost never entirely free from water. Even if they were, small amounts of moisture are usually introduced during processing or storage. The apparent solid state reactions leading to drug breakdown actually occur in a very thin layer of water adsorbed on the surface of drug crystals. There are a number of surprises encountered with solid dosage forms: putting certain drugs into gelatin capsules may lead to enormous stability problems even if the drugs are absolutely dry. The large amounts of moisture (15 per cent) in the gelatin shell may cause certain sensitive drugs to lose potency at a rapid rate.

When two finely divided powders are mixed and made into a tablet, the total surface of drug A in contact with drug B is about one square meter (approximately 1600 square inches). Deterioration in such a tablet would be very high if these were incompatible drugs. A significant improvement in the stability of the product may be achieved by reducing the area of contact between the two drugs. Making a two-layered tablet reduces the area of contact to less than one-half square inch. Separating the two drug layers by a layer of inactive materials further improves stability.

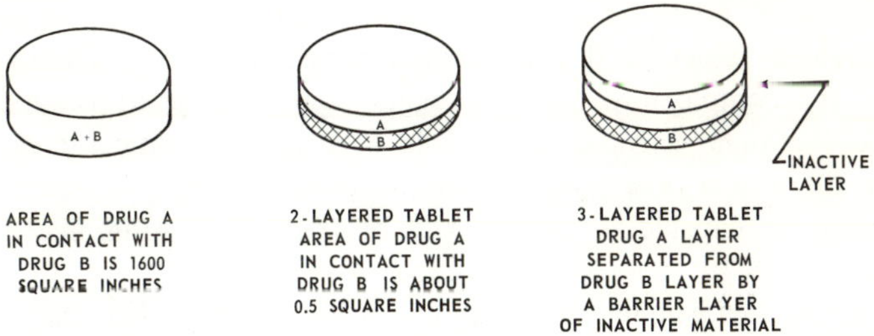

FIG. 35. Layered compressed tablets — a way of reducing area of contact between formulation components.

The triple-layer gives effective separation of the reactive drugs and usually improves the stability of the product. The possibility exists that reactive drug layers on different tablets may come into contact when the tablets are filled into a container. Generally, the contact is not sufficiently close to cause drug deterioration. If potency loss does occur, packaging of the tablets in plastic packets or strips may provide the needed additional protection. Compression or press-coated tablets represent another kind of solid dosage form capable of separating formulation components.

COMPRESSION COATED TABLET
CORE OF DRUG A COVERED
WITH COATING OF DRUG B

DOUBLE COMPRESSION
COATED TABLET
DRUG LAYERS SEPARATED
BY AN INACTIVE BARRIER COAT

FIG. 36. Compression coated tablets — a tablet within a tablet.

Layered tablets and press-coated tablets are good examples of the complexities and challenges facing the pharmaceutical development scientist in his role of balancing critical factors in the design of a product. The simplest system – a standard tablet or capsule – usually will be tried first. After accelerated stability testing, the simple system may prove to be inadequate. Solving the stability problem may then require changing the formula to make a layered tablet or a double-press-coated tablet. Often the formulation used in making a good standard tablet will not be suitable for the press-coated tablet – the different materials may not bond together. It must be shown that the new dosage form can be made in a reproducible way on full scale equipment and that its stability is satisfactory.

Separation of reactive components in drug formulations may also be achieved by making a pill of the sensitive drug and placing it into a capsule containing a powder mixture of the other drugs.

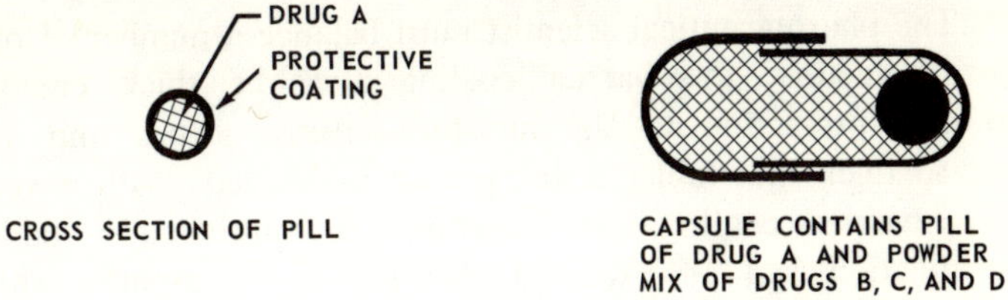

FIG. 37. Pills inside of capsules — a method of separating incompatible drugs.

Covering the pill with a protective coating effectively prevents contact between sensitive drug A and the other drugs. This kind of dosage form must be carefully checked to make certain that the protected drug will be released from the pill and produce the expected drug action when taken by the patient.

Vitamin products are unusually susceptible to deterioration or run-down in the presence of moisture. This is true even when they are put into tablets and capsules. Improved vitamin stability is obtained by coating the tablets with a moisture barrier and then with a sugar coating. Additional shelf-life may be achieved by using a barrier layer to separate one or more of the sensitive vitamins.

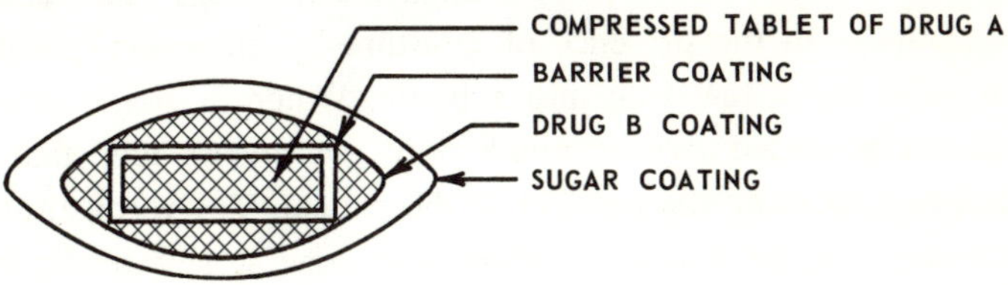

FIG. 38. A sugar coated tablet containing two incompatible drugs separated by a barrier layer.

The pharmaceutical scientist must balance a number of opposing factors: the barrier coating must be thick enough to give protection to the moisture-sensitive drugs and yet not so thick that tablet disintegration is delayed. With a very thin barrier coating, an experimental multivitamin tablet formulation had an expected shelf-life of 18 months when tested in an accelerated stability program. Disintegration time of this tablet in gastric juice was 30 minutes. Increasing the barrier coating improved the expected shelf life to 48 months but this also increased the disintegration time to 75 minutes. At first thought, the difference in time for the tablet to disintegrate does not seem very important; however, when the tablets were tested in human subjects, significant differences in the physiological availability of the vitamins were observed. The multivitamin tablet with the 75-minute disintegration time released less than 10 per cent of its riboflavin (Vitamin B_2) content for physiological absorption. In the same clinical test, the tablet with the 30-minute disintegration time delivered the riboflavin to the absorption sites in such a way that over 95 per cent was absorbed by the subject. Selecting a formula solely on the basis of superior stability is much like choosing a loaf of bread made from sawdust because it does not spoil!

Fluid products may be designed for drugs that easily decompose in the presence of moisture by filling dry powder or granules of the drug into a bottle. Water or some special diluent is added by the community pharmacist immediately before dispensing the product to the patient. The reconstituted product will be labeled to show how long it will retain full potency. Products of this kind must provide a significant advantage in storage quality in order to compensate for the disadvantage of the reconstitution step. Besides maintaining potency in the dry form, the granules should readily dissolve to form the desired, high quality, fluid product. A full potency lump in the bottom of the bottle obviously does not meet the quality requirements.

During the expected period of use, the reconstituted fluid product must retain at least 90 per cent of its labeled potency. For a drug that is stable in solution for 10 days, the largest package of the product would be one that is used up in this time. For example, at a dose of 3 teaspoons each day, the maximum package would be calculated as follows:

(3 teaspoons/day) x (5 milliliters/teaspoon) x 10 days = 150 milliliters (5 fluid ounces).

The Mix-O-Vial® represents a unique approach to the problem of achieving convenience and long storage at full potency. Relatively unstable drugs can be formulated without sacrificing the convenience factor. Components of the product are present in a single container but are separated by a rubber plug (see Fig. 39).

Pushing down on the top stopper results in the fluid transmitting the force to the center plug which is then pushed through. The fluid on top mixes with the powder in the bottom compartment — the preparation is ready for use. This system may be employed for oral fluid products; however, it finds greatest application for drugs administered by injection. For parenteral products, the bottom compartment of the vial may be filled with sterile drug powder or the powder added as a solution and the water removed by freeze-drying. Freezing the drug solution and evaporating or subliming away the water under high vacuum produces a porous cake that goes into solution very readily. After the bottom compartment is filled, frozen, and dried, the center plug is inserted. The

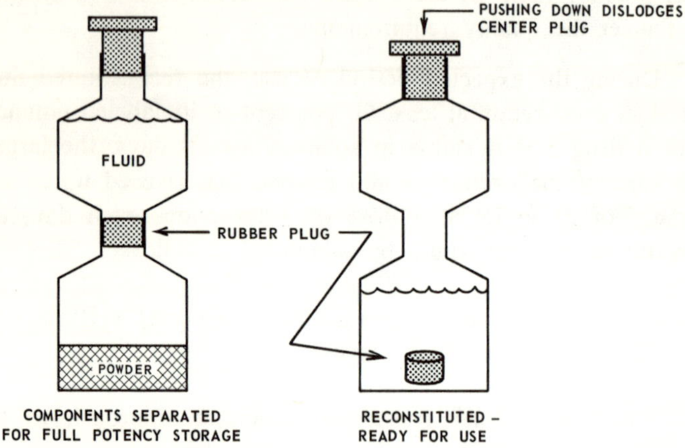

FIG. 39. The Mix-O-Vial® — a novel container for separating components of a fluid formulation until ready for use.

top compartment is then filled with diluent fluid under rigidly controlled sterile conditions. Designing superior products of this kind involves careful selection of formulation components and proper processing conditions — quality is achieved by careful balancing of all factors relating to the product.

BUGS

Pharmaceutical products must meet the highest standards for purity. Bugs — big and little — should not be present when the product is made nor should they be attracted to the product during storage. Big bugs or insects are relatively easy to keep out of the product — this requires good housekeeping during manufacturing. Suitable containers will prevent insect infestation during storage. Concern for the labeling is also in order if the product is to be stored in tropical climates — insects have been known to eat paper labels. Problems with big bugs are relatively easy to solve. Little bugs (bacteria and other micro-organisms) present a much greater problem to the development scientist. Micro-organisms are so small that they cannot be seen without a powerful microscope. They are found everywhere in enormous quantities within our natural environment. So prevalent are micro-organisms that their absence from an area or object is an unnatural condition — we speak of a sterile room or a sterile product, meaning that it is absolutely free from micro-organisms.

Products used in the eye and those used by injection must be sterile. This is an *absolute* requirement. The products must be free from micro-organisms and also free from cell fragments. The metabolic breakdown or waste products of bacterial growth must not be present in parenteral or injectable products.

Sterilization of liquid products may be accomplished by autoclaving or heating the product with steam under pressure (15 pounds of pressure at 121°C. for 20 minutes). Autoclaving is essentially the same as heating the product in a pressure cooker. This kind of sterilization of the product is fast and certain. It has an obvious drawback for drugs that are easily destroyed by heat. Special filters are available for sterilizing heat-sensitive products. The fluid product is put through the sterilizing filter under aseptic (germ-free) conditions, filled into sterile containers, and then sealed.

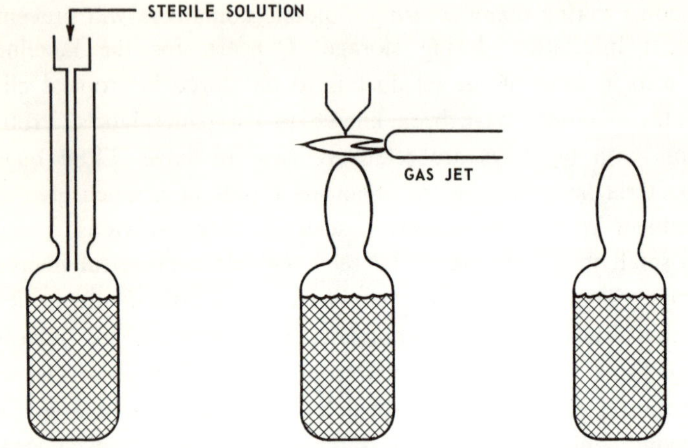

FIG 40. Ampul filling and sealing — basic steps for the single dose sterile product container.

In the single dose ampul, the product only touches glass. From the standpoint of stability, this gives the best protection. Drug solutions stored in ampuls will retain their sterility indefinitely so long as the container remains intact.

Containers holding two or more doses of a parenterally administered drug are called multiple dose vials. Products in multiple dose vials must also be sterile. In addition, they must contain chemical agents which preserve the sterility after the first dose is removed. When such preservatives are added, it is important that they do not lose their anti-microbial or preservative activity on storage. Therefore, it is necessary to carry out accelerated stability studies on the preservative as well as the active drug components of such products.

Selection of the closure may be a critical step in attaining good preservative activity in a multiple-dose injectable. Many preservatives are adsorbed from solution by certain kinds of rubber closures. Compatibility of the closure with the drug solution and with other components in the finished formula must be tested in a detailed and systematic fashion. A closure meeting all the conflicting requirements may well be thought of as an X-type essential component.

Eye drops present a special kind of challenge to the designer of such products. In normal usage, the dropper should not be allowed to touch the infected eye. This may, of course, happen inadvertently and cause the remaining doses of the product to become contaminated. For this reason, ophthalmic or eye products must not support microbial growth. Ideally, these dosage forms should be self-sterilizing. Selection of a good preservative for an experimental eye drop formulation is not easy — the requirements are very stringent. The preservative must be compatible with the drug, other formulation components, and the container. The preservative must be safe for inflamed or sensitive eyes, and it must retain its preservative activity against a variety of micro-organisms for the life of the product. For each experimental formulation, it is necessary to conduct microbiological tests to prove the effectiveness of the proposed preservative against various micro-organisms. Accelerated stability tests must be conducted with the best preserved experimental formulations to make certain that both drug and preservative activity are maintained during storage. Finally, the experimental formulations must be tested in rabbits for possible eye irritation prior to selecting the best formula for clinical testing in humans.

Fluid drug products intended for oral administration require preservatives to prevent spoilage due to mold and bacterial growth. Even fluid antibiotic products are susceptible to this kind of spoilage — certain micro-organisms are resistant to antibiotics and will grow in the presence of high concentrations of the drug. Many fluid products require several kinds of preservatives each having different anti-microbial activities. Using two preservatives gives added protection against the rare but troublesome kind of micro-organism that grows in the presence of one preservative. Some micro-organisms produce enzymes capable of destroying a single preservative — added reason to use more than one.

Seeding tests are generally carried out on all formulations containing preservatives. This involves the addition of large quantities of micro-organisms to samples of the experimental formulations. The samples are then kept under conditions favorable to microbial growth. In this manner, the over-all effectiveness of the preservative in the formulation is tested under the extreme circumstance of gross microbial contamination. The preservative must do more than retard or restrict growth of micro-organisms: it must not alter the chemical or physical properties of the product. A balancing of the factors of preservative selection must include concern for the effect on the taste of the product and the effectiveness of its drug content.

CHAPTER IV

Performance

SAFETY FIRST

THE DESIGNER of a pharmaceutical product must balance many diverse factors to achieve the best possible drug formulation and most effective dosage form. Experimental formulations are constantly evaluated and modified during the early development phase in a systematic search for the optimum combination of ingredients or conditions of manufacture. Ideally, the designer would like to have a formulation with maximum shelf life that can be manufactured at the minimum cost. In practice, this is only rarely achieved — some trade-offs are necessary. In the over-all process of designing the optimum formulation, the safety factor must never be compromised.

To the designer of pharmaceutical products, safety is one of the most important performance qualities. Product safety means that the finished formulation must be no less safe than the drug it contains. The various ingredients added to the formulation to improve stability, acceptability, and effectiveness of the drug component must — singly and in combination — be at least as safe as the drug itself. These "inactive" ingredients should not intensify the inherent toxicity of the drug. It is important to understand that safety is a relative term. There is, of course, no such thing as absolute drug safety. Misuse of any drug by overdosing or prolonged use without medical supervision may have serious consequences.

The safety check of an experimental formulation is done first in animals. For comparison purposes, a base line must be established with the simplest possible system. This is usually a solution of drug in water with no other materials present. In acute toxicity studies, the drug is administered to different species of animals in increasingly large doses. The drug would be administered at a given dose level to ten animals (rats or mice). The dose of the drug is always administered on the basis of body weight. Initially, this would be at a low dose of, say, 100 milligrams of drug per kilogram of animal weight. At these starting doses with a given drug, perhaps one out of ten animals would die. The experiment is repeated with another group of ten animals at a dose level of 200 milligrams of drug per kilogram of body weight with the result that three out of ten animals die. Increasing doses are given to groups of animals until nine out of ten or ten out of ten die. From such toxicity studies, the dose of pure drug which will cause death 50 per cent of the time in a given species of animals is calculated. This value is known as the LD_{50} (lethal dose — 50 per cent); the method of dose administration (oral, intravenous) and the species of animal are specified. In general, the higher the LD_{50}, the safer the drug. However, the dose of the drug required for a therapeutic effect must also be considered. Ideally, the curative dose of the drug is small, say, 10mg./kg., and the lethal dose is large (1000 mg./kg.) — the difference is the margin of safety.

Formulation ingredients and the method of manufacture may improve the effectiveness of a drug product by increasing shelf life or providing better dose uniformity. Each added ingredient should perform its intended function without hindering the performance of the drug or the other additives. In practice, of course, this is not always the case. The more components there are present in a formulation, the greater will be the likelihood of unwanted interactions. Checking the performance of the system is an important part of product design. This becomes increasingly difficult to do as the complexity of the system increases. As a general rule, the number of components in the formulation is kept at the minimum needed to do the job. Each ingredient should be present for a specific purpose and only in required amounts. For example, the amount of preservative present in an injectable product should be the minimum needed to provide protection with a reasonable margin of safety.

Selecting formulation components involves an intricate balancing process to meet the requirements of an effective, stable, satisfying, and economical product. Design of a balanced formula begins with the assembly of all available information on the chemical and physical properties of the components. Compatibility of the formulation ingredients is essential to ensure reliable drug release and maintain potency over long periods. Above all, the product must be safe! Safety of the formulation begins with its component parts. Materials used in drug products must first be tested extensively in animals to prove that they are safe. This kind of information is known as toxicology data.

The first function of the container is to protect the product. Physical and chemical stability of the formulation should be maintained at optimum levels for the product's expected shelf life. Consumer acceptance of the product may depend on the appeal or convenience factors of the container. Additionally, the container must not alter the safety or performance of the product. The problem of product safety and performance in various kinds of containers has been studied very intensively since plastic containers have become more common. The problem is particularly difficult because there are so many kinds of plastics. Even those containers made from the same plastic may differ significantly in over-all composition.

Plastic containers are generally not composed of a single pure material — additives are combined with plastics to aid in molding the containers to provide stability against light and oxygen, and to provide proper hardness. Some plastics may contain five or more different components each of different chemical reactivity. It is not surprising, then, that the selection of a plastic container requires a great deal more testing than is the case with glass containers. Safety of plastic containers must be established before they are used with drug products. After the product has been formulated, its stability in glass containers is determined. This provides base line information for selecting an appropriate plastic container. Tests with the final formula must be conducted to make certain that the plastic container does not affect the contents and that the contents do not affect the container. It is especially important to make certain that the components of the plastic do not combine with the drug or additives to form toxic compounds.

TEST TUBE TESTS

Product performance is achieved by an uncompromising concern for quality. The standards of quality designed into the product must be maintained through the years that the product is manufactured. The dosage form must maintain its full drug potency under normal storage conditions for the period of time indicated by the expiration dating. The product also must retain the same consumer appeal as when it was first made. All these aspects of the product quality must be carefully defined — values of acceptable ranges must be expressed in numbers. To ensure that each finished product meets high quality standards, properly designed tests are conducted during processing and in a final control check before the product is released for sale.

Complex systems such as suspensions of a solid drug in a flavored fluid offer special challenges to the development scientist in designing tests to predict long term physical stability. Simple accelerated stability tests at higher temperatures may not always give reliable predictions. Under actual storage conditions, the drug product may be subjected to alternating cycles of heat and cold. Crystals of the suspended drug may tend to grow under just the right conditions of heating and cooling to produce a mass of large crystals that cannot be resuspended for uniform dosing. When this happens, the customer will be very unhappy — the product will not be purchased a second time.

Performance tests conducted in the laboratory must be checked periodically against actual use conditions. The correlation first established during the development phase of a new product may not provide reliable predictions of product performance if a number of changes have been introduced into the manufacturing process. Changes may be so gradual as to be almost unnoticed. For example, machine improvements may increase the speed of a tablet packaging machine by 40 per cent over a period of five years. The laboratory test measuring the resistance of the tablets to breaking and abrasion would show no change in the tablet characteristics from those of the first production batch. Under actual use conditions, the tablets would show more breakage than that predicted by the quality control test. When this happens, the control test must be improved to give better prediction and the quality of the product must be improved to give better performance.

Time changes the standards of quality — ever upward. Each time one of the factors affecting quality is changed, all factors must be redetermined. The development scientist must be prepared to rebalance the factors of stability, consumer acceptance, economic return, and the drug availability when altering the factor of production feasibility. Maintaining the quality of a pharmaceutical product is an expensive operation!

Ideally, products should be designed to be as foolproof as possible under all conditions of manufacturing, storage, and use. The development scientist must have on hand all pertinent information about actual conditions under which the product is to be manufactured. This is especially important if it is to be made in foreign countries. Storage conditions may be vastly different for products shipped into international areas. The development scientist who designs drug products for world-wide use must contend with as many factors as a military leader equipping an army to fight in both the frozen arctic and in tropical jungles.

ROCKETS AND TABLETS

Dosage forms and ballistic missiles have much in common — both are delivery systems. Their effectiveness does not depend solely on how much is in them — a vehicle is judged on whether or not it gets to where it is supposed to go. Delivery of contents is the critical test of performance. Tablets are the means by which a measured dose of drug is delivered to the target site — the area in the gastrointestinal (G.I.) tract where drug absorption takes place. During storage the tablet must protect the drug from deterioration. When taken by the patient, the tablet must rapidly disintegrate into small pieces. The drug in the pieces or granules must dissolve and be in solution at the site in the gastrointestinal tract where absorption takes place.

Since the tablet must disintegrate when taken, one of the routine laboratory tests involves evaluation of this property. During the development of the tablet formula, the tablet disintegration test is used to select the formulation giving the most reproducible and, generally, the shortest disintegration time. This test plays an important part in controlling the tablet quality during manufacture. The test information is used to make certain that each lot performs the same as the original with respect to disintegration into granules.

The tablet disintegration test is conducted under carefully controlled conditions in a specially designed apparatus. The essential features of this test are shown in Figure 41.

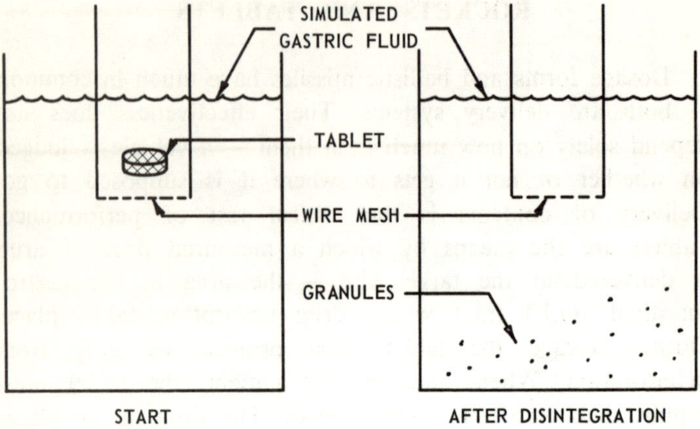

FIG. 41. The tablet disintegration test.

The tablet to be tested is placed in a glass tube having a wire mesh bottom. This basket-like arrangement is mechanically agitated at a controlled rate in the test fluid. Temperature is maintained at 37°C. (body temperature) during the test. Disintegration of the tablet is taken as the time when substantially all of the tablet passes through the screen.

Tablet disintegration is important because it is the first step in the essential sequence affecting drug performance:

(1) Tablet Disintegrates (2) Drug in Granules Dissolves (3) Drug is Absorbed

Rapid disintegration of the tablet does not ensure that the drug will go into solution. A tablet may disintegrate quite rapidly, say, in three minutes, but not release the drug to solution. If the drug does not dissolve at a reasonable rate in gastrointestinal fluids, it will not be absorbed. When this happens, the tablet will have failed in its primary mission of delivering the drug to the target site where absorption takes place.

Determining the dissolution characteristics of the drug component of a tablet requires a great deal more effort than does the determination of tablet disintegration time. A reliable assay procedure — a method for quantitative chemical analysis — is needed to measure the amount of drug released to solution. A single chemical analysis or assay may require one hour of a chemical technician's time. This would give a one point determination — we would have information about how much drug is released after, say, 15 minutes in the fluid. We would not know how much drug had been released after 5 minutes or 10 minutes. More information is needed to be certain that the tablet releases all of its drug content in a steady, predictable fashion. This requires additional chemical analyses or assays of the fluid during the course of a tablet dissolution test to establish a profile as shown in Figure 42.

Even ten separate assays might not entirely describe the dissolution profile. Filling in the gaps would, of course, improve the information about the experimental formulations. Obtaining more data is always a very costly operation. In every development program, the decision on information must be made: *how* much to assemble of *what* kind and *when*. Often this decision must be made on a daily basis. Certainly, it is always desirable to have all of the data that *might* apply to the project. This is only rarely achieved. One point is always before us: information costs time and money! The development scientist must make the decision many times in each project on whether to study one part more intensively or to go on to the next phase. His technical judgment also dictates how much time and effort should be spent in putting

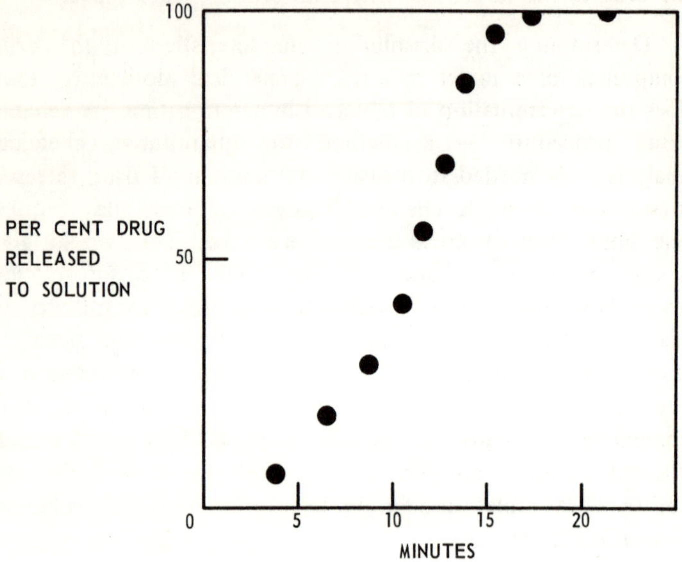

FIG. 42. Tablet dissolution test — a profile of drug released to solution as a function of time.

parts of the project together in a complete package. Sound technical judgment usually makes the difference between having a pile of interesting reports and having a successful completed project.

HOSTILE ENVIRONMENT

Orally administered drugs must pass through the stomach on their journey to absorption sites in the intestinal tract.

Some drugs are absorbed through the walls of the stomach but most are absorbed in the upper part of the small intestine called the duodenum. The stomach presents a hostile environment to certain kinds of acid-sensitive drugs.

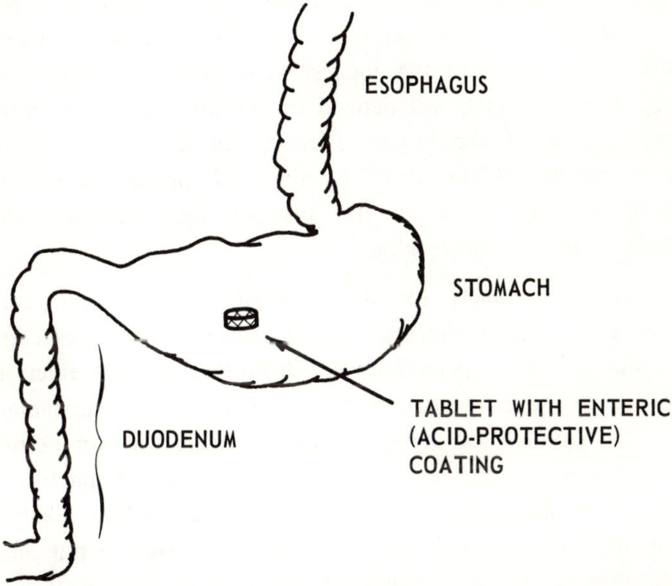

FIG. 43. The environment in which oral dosage forms operate as drug delivery systems.

The stomach functions as a container for holding food until it is ready to proceed through the digestive system. Some processing of the food does take place to prepare it for later absorption from the intestine. Chewed food is churned in the stomach in the presence of gastric fluid, a strongly acidic composition of dilute hydrochloric acid and the enzymes pepsin, rennin, and lipase. In the holding process, proteins are broken down to amino acids; fats are reduced to small particles and partially converted; carbohydrates are not much affected. The rate of emptying the stomach is greatly dependent upon the composition of food put into it: carbohydrates are released faster than proteins while fatty meals are held the longest. The residence time of a drug in the stomach will depend on the kind of dosage form used and all of the factors affecting the emptying time of the stomach. If the drug is absorbed mainly from the duodenum, the delay in the stomach may influence the efficiency of drug absorption.

Designing tablets for drugs sensitive to stomach acid requires great care: the drug must be given enough protection without affecting performance. Protection of a tablet is usually achieved by coating it with special polymeric materials. Such enteric or acid-protecting coatings will not permit drug release in the acid environment of the stomach but will allow the tablet to disintegrate in the mildly alkaline conditions of the duodenum. The amount of coating put onto the tablet is extremely critical. If too little is used, protection against stomach acid will not be sufficient and drug deterioration will occur before absorption takes place. If too much coating is used, the tablet may not disintegrate until it is well past the site of absorption. Balancing the factors to arrive at the proper level and kind of coating requires a knowledge of coating technology and a thorough understanding of gastro-intestinal physiology.

CONTROLLING RELEASE

Tablets may be designed to release their drug content uniformly over a long period of time rather than in the off-on fashion of enteric-coated tablets. Prolonging the release of drug may be desired in order to achieve a more convenient dosing schedule. The controlled drug release from solid dosage forms is accomplished by properly combined components. Ingredients added for this purpose are the most important kind of X-type ingredients — performance of the product as a drug delivery system is altered.

Designing a sustained or prolonged action product requires a great deal of information about the biological and chemical properties of the drug. Important biological properties that must be known about the drug include the dose-activity relationship and the toxicity pattern; information must also be available on the rate processes of drug absorption, distribution, metabolism, and excretion. Solubility of the drug and its chemical reactivity are just a few of the physical-chemical properties that must be taken into account when designing the dosage form.

One of the interesting approaches to the problem of providing sustained drug action involves combining the drug with a finely powdered plastic-like or polymeric material and forming the mixture into a tablet. The polymer selected for this purpose should have a low solubility in gastrointestinal fluids and should not react with the drug nor bind it in such a way that it cannot all get out of the tablet. An additional important requirement for the polymer is that it should be physiologically inactive — that is, it should possess no drug activity of its own. Tablets containing a drug mixed with an insoluble polymer possess a matrix structure in that most of the drug particles are surrounded by polymer particles.

Sustained action is obtained by the drug slowly dissolving or leaching out of the matrix tablet. The matrix-type tablet does not readily disintegrate. When all of the drug has dissolved from the tablet, a soft sponge-like skeleton of the insoluble plastic matrix remains behind. The matrix presents a kind of maze through which the dissolved drug molecules must pass to reach the fluids outside of the tablet. The pathway traveled through the tablet is longer than it is in the case of regular tablets. Conventional compressed tablets break up or disintegrate into small granules, thereby exposing much more surface to dissolution fluids. The disintegration process also effectively shortens the distance for diffusion. In the matrix-type tablet, the time required for the drug molecule to make the transit to the tablet surface is increased.

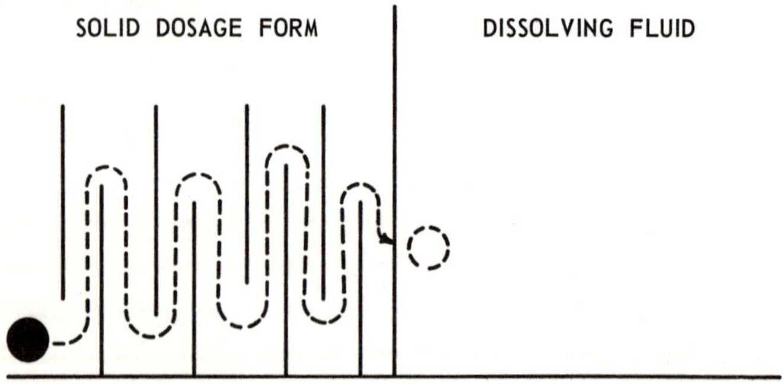

FIG. 44. Matrix tablets present a twisted pathway for diffusing drug molecules.

Dissolved drug molecules move by diffusion through calm, unstirred fluid inside the wetted tablet. When the dissolved drug molecules reach the surface of the tablet, the stirring action of the gastrointestinal tract helps sweep them away from the surface of the tablet. The dissolved drug molecules are then mixed with the bulk of the gastrointestinal fluid and move to the site of absorption.

DRUG (SOLID) IN TABLET

↓ STEP 1

DRUG (DISSOLVED) IN TABLET

↓ STEP 2

DRUG (DISSOLVED) IN FLUID NEXT TO TABLET SURFACE

↓ STEP 3

DRUG (DISSOLVED) AT SITE OF INTESTINAL ABSORPTION

↓ STEP 4

DRUG (DISSOLVED) ABSORBED AND DISTRIBUTED IN BODY

FIG. 45. Drug absorption from a matrix tablet — a sequence of steps.

If diffusion within the tablet is slow, this means that the rate at which dissolved drug molecules reach the surface of the tablet will likewise be slow. Diffusion may be the slowest or rate-determining step in the over-all process of drug absorption from a tablet. By controlling the diffusion step, it is possible to control drug release.

Coatings may be applied to conventional compressed tablets to produce dosage forms with prolonged or sustained drug release characteristics. The polymeric materials used for such coating are not sensitive to changes in the acidity of gastrointestinal contents. In this respect, they differ from enteric coatings. Coatings for prolonged drug release act as barriers to the wetting of the drug in the tablet; these coatings also slow the outward diffusion of dissolved drug molecules. More importantly, the intact coating holds the tablet together, preventing its break up into small granules. This means that the surface of the tablet exposed to the bulk fluid in the gastrointestinal tract will remain constant. As in the case of the matrix tablet, almost no stirring takes place within the tablet — release of the drug remains essentially constant from such systems.

ABSORPTION

Product performance must be judged on an objective basis. It is not enough to say that the formula is "better than," we must be able to say better than *what* and by *how much*. In order to do this, we must have a valid base line for comparing performance. The base line or comparison standard for dosage forms should be drug absorption from the simplest system of all — an aqueous solution of the drug.

Designing an effective dosage form requires an intimate knowledge of the factors affecting drug absorption, distribution, metabolism and excretion. Blood is the distribution system of the body. When an orally administered drug is absorbed from the gastrointestinal tract, it is carried by the blood to the site of action. The concentration in the blood following an oral dose is shown as an idealized curve.

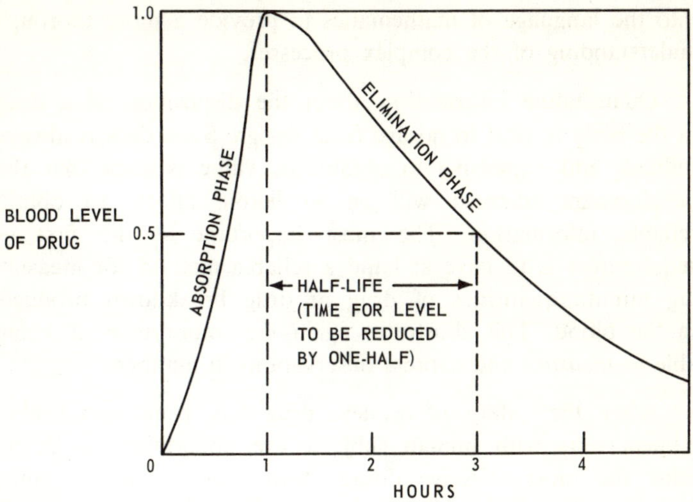

FIG. 46. Blood level of a drug following an oral dose given as a solution.

The blood level-time plot is of importance in understanding the way a drug acts in the body. Drug activity is an ever-changing, dynamic process — time is always a factor in drug performance. The time activity relationship is greatly influenced by design characteristics of the dosage form. In order to evaluate the effectiveness of experimental dosage forms, it is necessary to know the rate of drug absorption and excretion in the absence of formulation influences. The drug excretion or elimination phase occurs after the peak blood level. It is described in terms of the time period required for the blood level of drug to be reduced by one-half — the so-called biological half-life. In the actual process of designing dosage forms, graphic information of the kind shown in the above blood level-time plot must be translated into the language of mathematics to provide a more thorough understanding of the complex processes.

Quantitative information about the disposition of a drug in the body is vital to dosage from design. Such data is always difficult and expensive to obtain; its value is such that the development scientist will go to heroic efforts to obtain reliable information. The most important — the first — requirement is to have at hand a reliable method for measuring minute quantities of drug or drug breakdown products in the blood. This illustrates again the importance of being able to *measure* and express observations in numbers.

After the safety of a new drug has been established, clinical tests with human subjects are undertaken to determine the most effective dosage form. Before this is done, it is usually helpful if some of the preliminary drug availability experiments can be carried out in animals. Dosage form evaluation in animals presents the advantage of obtaining a lot of information in a reasonable time at a minimum cost. It is not, however, free from disadvantages! Different animal species show widely varying patterns of drug absorption. This is especially true for orally administered drugs which must be absorbed from the gastrointestinal tract.

Comparing the efficiency of two different dosage forms of a drug in a test animal presents many difficulties. Consider the case of an experimental coated tablet 9 millimeters (about 1/3 inch) in diameter containing 100 milligrams of drug A. Assume this is the average dose of this drug for an adult weighing 70 kilograms (154 lb.). Testing the intact tablets in rats would be out of the question — the dosage forms would be too big for the rat to swallow. A larger animal like a dog would be able to swallow the intact tablet but the results of such a test would be highly questionable. Giving the 100 milligram tablet to a 7 kilogram dog would be a ten-fold overdose of drug. Beside the possible toxic reaction, the high dose might be absorbed differently than a normal dose. The simple expedient would seem to be to break the tablet and administer a tiny piece corresponding to the proper dose. This, of course, would destroy the integrity of the coated tablet — the drug release characteristics of the whole tablet may be significantly different from that of small pieces.

LITTLE PILLS

Miniaturization of dosage forms has been used by pharmaceutical scientists in their efforts to obtain reliable estimates of performance in animals. Tiny tablets one-tenth the over-all dimensions of a standard tablet have been made for administering drug to small animals in dosage form comparison studies. These tiny tablets have been coated with the same sort of protective and controlled release coatings used for standard tablets. In this way, the composition of the test dosage form can be kept identical to that of the intact, full-scale tablet. Even with this sort of special planning, some inherent difficulties are encountered in evaluating oral dosage forms in animals. For example, the differences in the acidity of the stomach juices of small animals make evaluation of enteric-coated tablets particularly difficult.

The speed with which fluid contents are moved through the gastrointestinal tract differs greatly in various animals. This may result in the test dosage form being propelled past the site of absorption before complete disintegration and dissolution can take place. If the drug in a tablet or granule goes into solution after the tablet has passed the primary site of absorption, not much of the dose will be absorbed. The resultant blood level will likely be quite low. This would indicate that the dosage form is not an effective drug delivery system — for that animal species. It is generally necessary to check performance in several species of animals using appropriately designed miniature dosage forms. The scientific design of dosage forms can be greatly aided by using animal tests for preliminary evaluations. Of course, the final performance test of the dosage form is the way it works as a drug delivery system in man.

CROSSOVER TESTS

The concept of *crossover* is critical to dosage form comparison studies. Simply put, crossover means that each animal or subject would receive each kind of dosage form so that a fair comparison can be made. Consider the case of two dosage forms A and B each containing the same drug but combined in different formulations. These are to be evaluated by comparing the resultant blood levels when administered to Subjects 1 and 2. A *simple* comparison would involve giving A to Subject 1 and B to Subject 2. Results of the comparison study might show significantly higher blood levels obtained with dosage form A. The difference might be due to the fact that Subject 1 was a better absorber of the drug. This subject might exhibit higher blood levels no matter what dosage form is used. Administering A to both Subject 1 and Subject 2 on one day and then giving B to both on another day provides a better comparison. Such an experiment does not take into account the possibility that both subjects may exhibit lower than normal responses on the second trial due to conditions not related to dosage form B. For example, the prior test with dosage form A may alter the response to the drug given in dosage form B. Slight changes in the subjects' diet on the day of the second test may have a profound effect on the performance of the dosage form. The *crossover* design provides for an objective and bias-free comparison:

	Subject 1	Subject 2
Day 1	A	B
Day 7	B	A

For a two-way crossover experiment with larger numbers of subjects, half would receive preparation A and half preparation B on each test day; test days would be spaced to prevent prior testing from influencing results.

The blood level produced by administering a drug in solution provides an objective comparison standard against which the drug delivery efficiency of an experimental dosage form may be compared as indicated in Figure 47.

Results of such comparisons, conducted under crossover conditions, provide the basis for the pharmaceutical scientist's decision to improve the experimental formulation. In this way, additional work on the efficiency of the drug delivery system would be guided by objective measurement of performance — blood levels.

The dosage form must provide the proper protection for the drug which it contains. The dosage form must be suitable for full-scale production at a reasonable cost. Above all, the dosage form must provide reproducible and effective drug

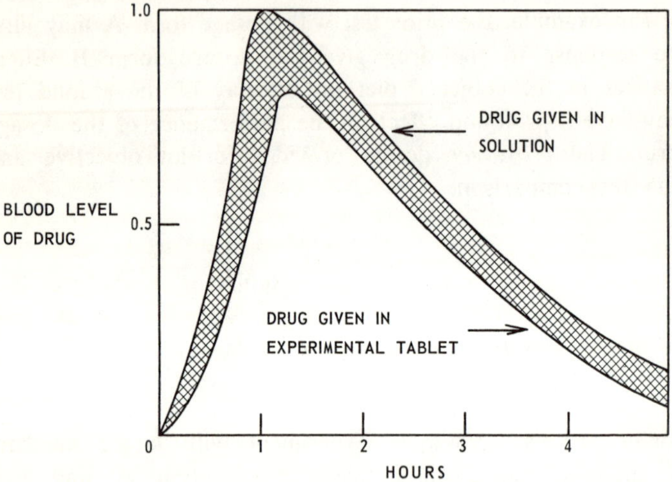

FIG 47. Comparative blood levels produced by equivalent doses of a drug given as a solution and as an experimental tablet.

absorption. Systematic selection and evaluation of formula components is an essential part of the designing of a superior dosage form — each non-drug ingredient becomes an ingredient X. The balancing of factors requires, in each case, checking the effect on the whole system. Again, we see the importance of measurement to the scientist in his work. Without measurement there is no such thing as applied science — only art.

Design of injectable products involves the selection of formulation components or additives to ensure product stability and sterility. In addition, it must be conclusively demonstrated that the additives do not impair the performance of the product as a drug delivery system. If an experimental parenteral product is injected into muscle, it is obvious that the total dose is put into the body. However, the rate at which the drug is absorbed from the injection site may be dependent on the composition of the formulation. The time that it takes for the blood level to fall to one-half its original value (half-life or *t*-50 per cent) in the elimination phase gives a measure of the rate or velocity of drug elimination. Comparing the half-life obtained with intramuscular (I.M.) and intravenous (I.V.) injections provides important information about the performance of an experimental injectable product.

A scientific approach to dosage form design requires information about the absorption, distribution, metabolism, and excretion of the drug. Sometimes, it happens that this information is almost unattainable because conventional chemical and physical methods of analysis cannot measure drug at the concentrations present in the body. For example, a potent drug given in a dose of 1 milligram (0.001 gram) when uniformly distributed throughout the body of an average man weighing 70 kilograms will be present in blood at a concentration of:

$$\frac{1.0 \times 10^{-3} \text{ grams of drug}}{70. \times 10^{3} \text{ grams of body weight}} = \begin{array}{l}1.43 \times 10^{-8} \text{ grams of drug} \\ \text{per gram or milliliter} \\ \text{of body tissue or fluid.}\end{array}$$

Each milliliter of blood would contain *0.0000000143 grams of drug*. If we assume that the most sensitive available method of analysis requires a sample containing 0.0002 grams of drug for reliable measurement, we can calculate the corresponding volume of blood needed:

$$\frac{2 \times 10^{-4} \text{ grams of drug}}{1.43 \times 10^{-8} \text{ grams of drug/ml. of blood}} = 1.4 \times 10^{4} \text{ or } 14{,}000 \text{ milliliters of blood.}$$

This would indicate at once the need for a much more sensitive assay — there just isn't that much blood in a person! The average blood volume is about 8 per cent of body weight or 5600 milliliters for a person weighing 70 kilograms. Actually, most drugs are not uniformly distributed throughout the body but are concentrated in the different organs. Volumes of distribution of a number of drugs vary from that of total blood volume to about 20,000 milliliters.

RADIOACTIVE LABELS

Measuring minute quantities of drug in biological fluids is much like trying to find and count needles in a haystack. The need for reliable methods of drug analysis has prompted pharmaceutical scientists to explore the use of radio-active drugs for this purpose. Drugs labeled or "tagged" with radioactive carbon atoms may be measured quantitatively even in very small concentrations by using a radio activity measuring device like the Geiger Counter. Labeled drug molecules are specially made or synthesized from fragments containing the radioactive atoms.

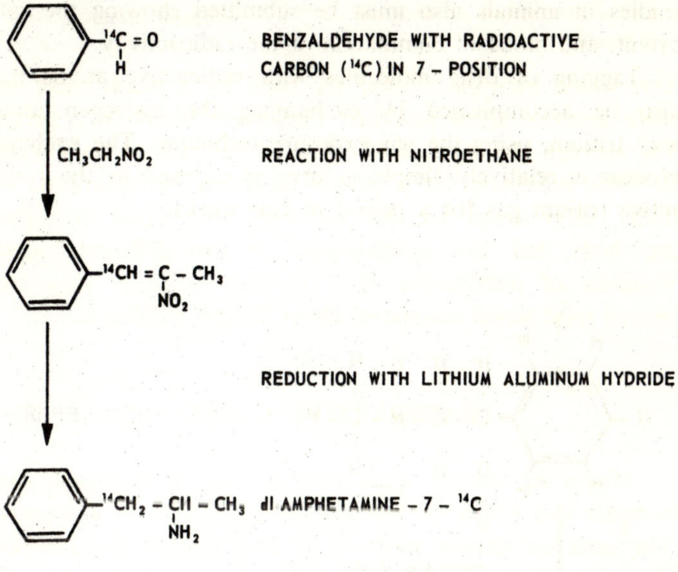

FIG. 48. Synthesis of the drug amphetamine with radioactive carbon atom (^{14}C) in a specific location.

Administration of a drug "tagged" with radioactive carbon does not endanger the health of the subjects. Radiocarbon (^{14}C) is a relatively weak beta ray emitter — only low levels of radiation are involved in such studies. There must be ample evidence on hand to show that the radioactive material will be completely eliminated from the body within a reasonably short time. The use of radioactive materials for drug absorption studies must be approved by the Atomic Energy Commission (AEC). Full disclosure of each proposed experiment must be made to the AEC, including the number of subjects, the kind and amount of radioactive materials and the qualifications of the investigators. Results of similar studies in animals also must be submitted showing the rate, extent, and mode of elimination of the radioactivity.

Tagging of drug molecules with radioactive atoms may also be accomplished by exchanging the hydrogen atoms with tritium, using the gas exposure technique. The exchange process is relatively simple — drug is exposed to the radioactive tritium gas for a period of two weeks.

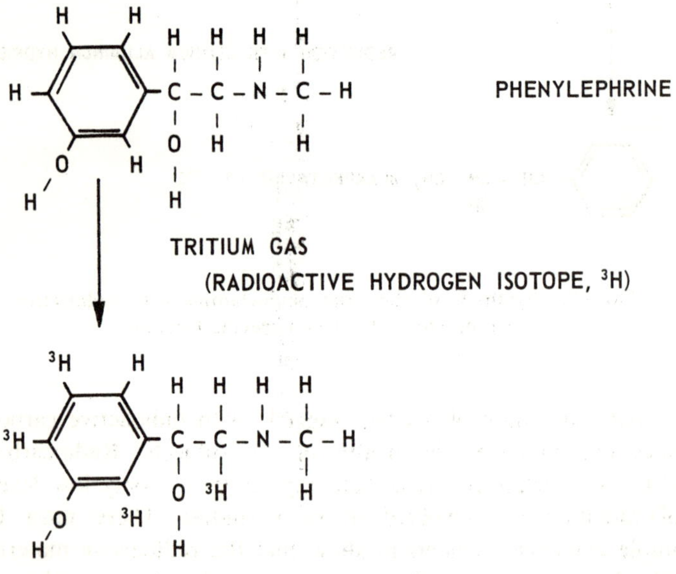

FIG. 49. Labeling the drug phenylephrine with tritium (^3H) — a random process for introducing radioactivity into the molecule.

The tritium replaces hydrogen atoms on the molecule in a random fashion. After the exchange reaction, the weakly bound tritium is removed by exposing the tritiated product to water. The tritiated product containing strongly bound tritium atoms is then purified. Tritium is the radioactive isotope of hydrogen; it differs from hydrogen in that there are two neutrons in the tritium nucleus — the nuclear instability results in the emission of weakly energetic beta rays. Tritium possesses the same chemical reactivity as does hydrogen — drug molecules containing tritium in place of hydrogen behave just like non-radioactive drugs.

In a typical kind of study, the radioactive drug is made into different tablet dosage forms, each containing the same dose of drug representing 100 microcuries of radioactivity. Determining the relative efficiency of the experimental tablet formulations involves administration to human subjects in a crossover experiment according to the following plan:

	Subject 1	Subject 2	Subject 3
Day 1	Tablet A	Tablet B	Tablet C
Day 10	Tablet B	Tablet C	Tablet A
Day 20	Tablet C	Tablet A	Tablet B

Each of the three subjects would receive, at different times, the three dosage forms. The 10-day interval between dosing ensures against cumulative drug or radioactivity effects. Samples of blood would be withdrawn at 30-minute intervals following administration of the dose. The level of radioactivity of each of the different blood samples is measured in a scintillation counter.

Scintillation counters depend on the fluorescence produced in certain liquids (phosphors) when irradiated. The radiation raises electrons in the phosphors to higher energy levels. When the electrons return to their normal or ground state, they emit light energy. The light flashes or scintillations are detected by a photomultiplier tube which converts the flashes into electrical pulses which are amplified and counted. Results of the radioactivity assay are reported as counts or disintegrations per minute (d.p.m.) per milliliter of blood plasma.

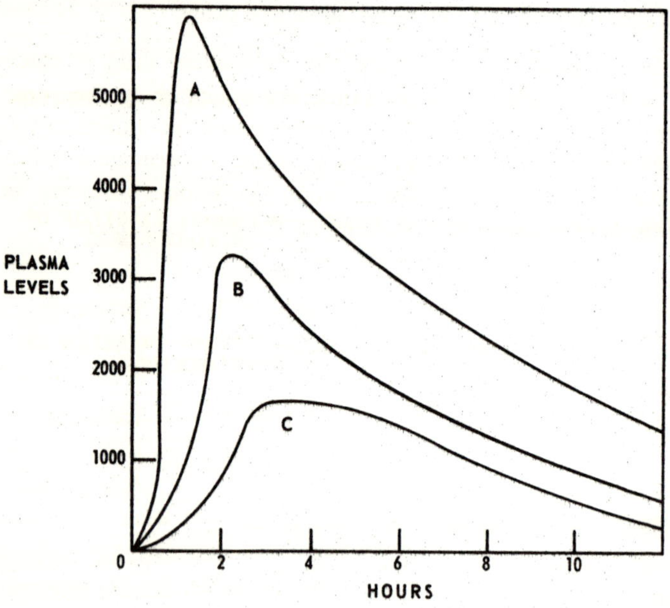

FIG. 50. Plasma levels of tritium radioactivity (disintegrations per minute per milliliter) following oral administration of identical doses of radioactive phenylephrine in different tablet formulations.

ACTIVITY AND RESPONSE

Drug response is related to drug activity or effective concentration: the higher the concentration of drug at the site of action, the greater the response. This does not necessarily mean that drug response will be directly proportional to drug concentration in the blood. The interrelationship of drug activity in the various compartments of the body is shown below:

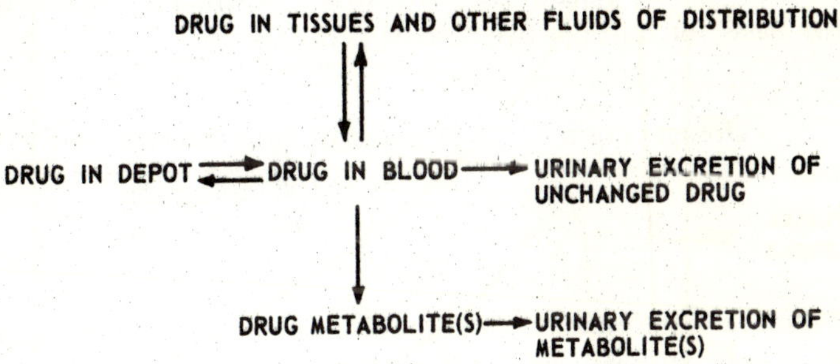

FIG. 51. Distribution of drug and metabolized drug in the body.

The distribution system is extremely complex. Doubling the concentration of drug in the blood does not result in an instantaneous doubling of activity in other compartments. The maximum concentration of drug at the site of action may lag behind the peak blood level.

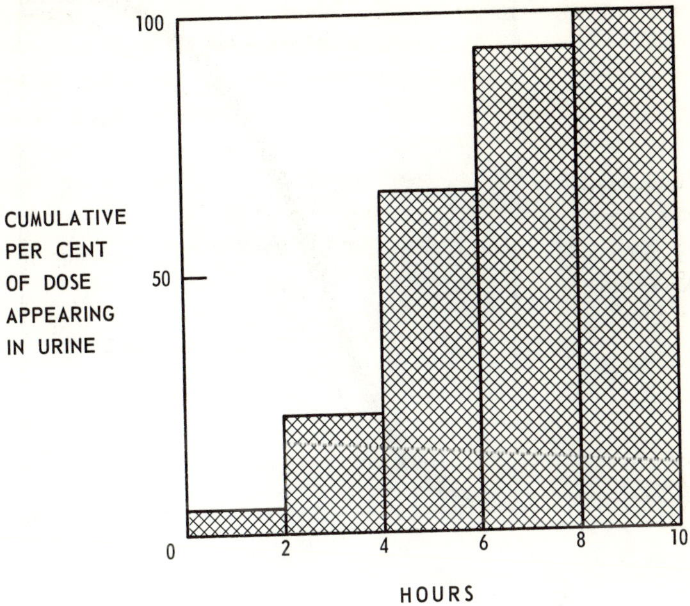

FIG. 52. Urinary excretion of drug in successive two hour periods — a cumulative bar graph representation.

Taking samples more frequently produces a smooth S-shaped curve. When urinary excretion data are plotted this way, appropriate mathematical expressions can be used to reproduce what the blood level curve would look like.

Urinary excretion data may be used to evaluate the efficiency of different experimental formulations.

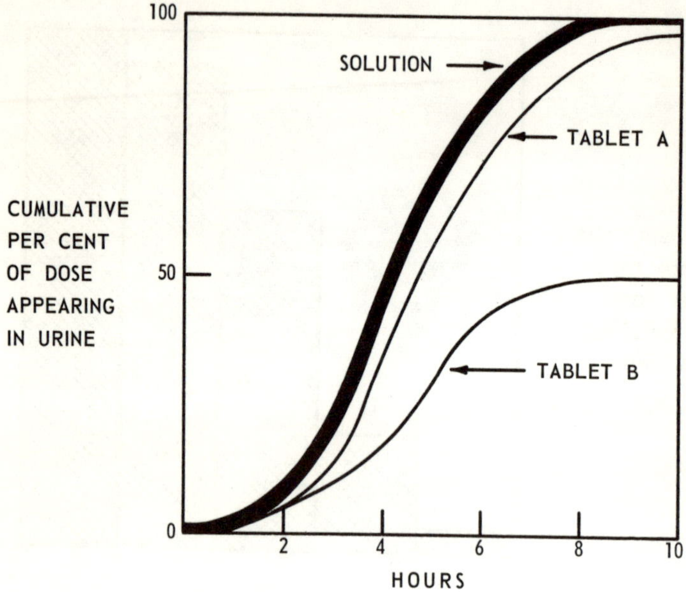

FIG. 53. Comparative plots of urinary excretion of drug when administered in solution and in two different tablet formulations.

Physiological availability of a drug from dosage forms is calculated by comparing the per cent of dose absorbed and subsequently excreted in the urine with values found after administration of the same dose in a standard preparation:

$$\% \text{ Availability} = \frac{\left(\begin{array}{l}\text{\% of Dose excreted} \\ \text{in a given time after taking test dosage form}\end{array}\right)}{\left(\begin{array}{l}\text{\% of Dose excreted in} \\ \text{same time after taking standard dosage form}\end{array}\right)} \times 100$$

Efficiency of dosage forms as drug delivery systems may also be measured by comparing the area under a blood level-time plot. This information tells us how much drug has been in the blood over a period of time. The area under a curve may be determined by drawing the figure on regular ruled graph paper and counting the squares or parts of squares under the line. For straight line geometric figures such as those shown in Figure 54, this is comparatively easy to do.

Actual blood level curves are only roughly approximated by straight line figures. Mathematically, the absorption and elimination phases are properly called first order processes because the rate of change is dependent on one variable — the concentration of drug. The logarithm of the blood level concentration plotted versus the time will give a straight line. On regular graph paper, blood level-time plots appear as shown in Figure 55.

The mathematical technique for determining the area under a curve is called integration. Using calculus, the precise area is found by filling it with rectangles of known area. Another approach to the problem of determining the area of non-linear figures is to use a planimeter — a simple instrument which measures area by passing a tracer wheel around the boundary line of the figure. For quick comparisons, the relative area of complex figures may be determined by drawing the figure on graph paper and then cutting out the figure and weighing it on an analytical balance. The relative areas of the shaded figures above were determined this way. Graph paper is surprisingly uniform in thickness — careful weighing can give estimates of area that differ from the true value by no more than 5 per cent.

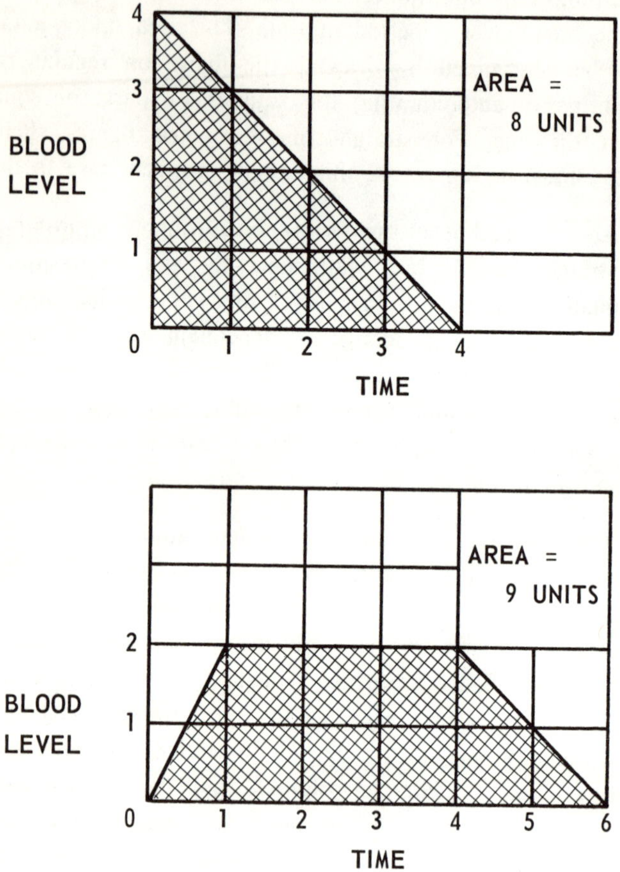

FIG. 54. Simplified examples of area measurements under blood level-time plots.

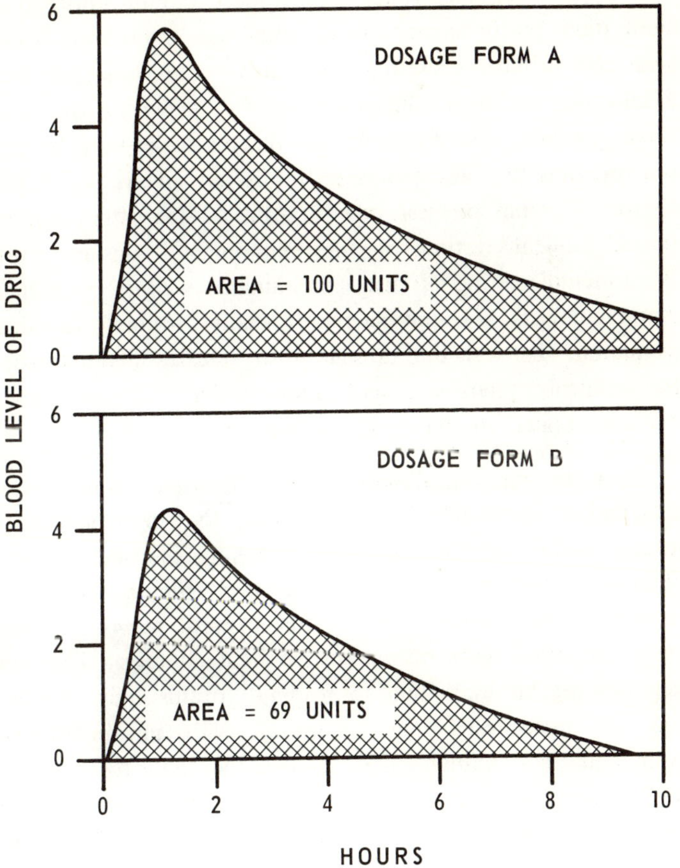

FIG. 55. Comparison of areas under blood level-time plots of identical doses of drug administered in two different dosage forms.

PLACEBO EFFECTS AND CLINICAL TESTS

The designer of dosage forms must obtain information about their performance under actual use conditions. Blood level and urinary excretion data provide an objective way of selecting the most efficient system for delivering the drug. While generally a safe assumption that the more rapid release rate provides the best response, this is not always so. Selecting the optimum or best rate of drug release often requires special clinical testing of the experimental dosage form. Experimental testing of drugs in humans is done by clinical pharmacologists — physicians specially trained in drug evaluation. To test the dosage form release characteristics, the clinical pharmacologist must select a measurable response related to the drug's activity.

Clinical pharmacologists have devised some very imaginative approaches for measuring the performance of dosage forms. Ideally, the act of making the measurement should not perturb the system nor affect the response. For example, drugs which act on the central nervous system affect an individual's response to a light stimulus. The time required for an individual to respond to this light stimulus may be measured quite accurately with an instrument. Stimulants like amphetamine shorten the time for response while central nervous system depressants like alcohol lengthen reaction time. The rate of drug release from the dosage form will influence the response pattern. The individual's response at any given time after taking the drug is compared to response under standard (no drug) conditions. The tests are carried out under "blind" conditions — the subject must not be able to tell from the appearance of the dosage form whether or not it contains drug. Designing the placebo dosage forms often proves to be as difficult as designing those with active drugs.

The controlled clinical experiment involves administration of a placebo (no drug) dosage form identical in appearance, taste, and odor to the drug dosage form. This is done to avoid the psychological response (the so-called placebo effect) to the act of taking a drug. In many cases, if a person receives a placebo capsule containing ordinary sugar and is told that it is a stimulant drug, he may report feeling stimulated. Most surprisingly, his heartbeat, blood pressure, and other vital signs might actually change as if he had been given a drug. Even without prompting by the clinical investigator, a test subject may, at times, report that a dosage form causes dizziness, nausea, or other side effects. Such comments may or may not be related to the drug or dosage form. The use of a placebo helps resolve this important question because the subject cannot distinguish the dosage form containing active drug. The clinical investigator is able to compare the results obtained with the placebo and the active drug dosage form in the same subject under identical conditions — this is the basic idea of a controlled experiment.

RECIPE FOR QUALITY

Selection of the optimum experimental formulation requires extreme diligence and the application of all relevant science and technology. The development job does not end there. The best of the formulations must be translated into a product that can be produced economically on a large scale while maintaining consistently high quality. The ultimate goal of the development scientist is to design a marketable new product of superior quality in the shortest possible time and at a reasonable cost.

Directions for making the new product must be written by the development scientist. This must be done in simple and clear language to avoid any possible misunderstandings. To do this, the development scientist must have a thorough knowledge of manufacturing equipment, practices and the training level of manufacturing personnel. Production of the high quality new product may require modification of equipment or a training program for plant operators. Quality doesn't just happen — it must be designed into the product and made an integral part of the manufacturing process.

Correlations between laboratory quality tests and product performance must be established during the development phase. The quality control tests should ensure that the product has the same performance characteristics as the original formulation made in the laboratory. The manufactured product should always correspond to the experimental or prototype formulation so carefully tested in the clinic. Correlations should cover a range of test values that might be encountered during manufacture. For example, the physiological availability of drug from a compressed tablet may show the following relationship to laboratory disintegration time and dissolution rate.

Tablet Disintegration Time	Time for 50% of Drug to Dissolve (t-50%)	Physiological Availability
3 minutes	4 minutes	100%
7	8	100%
10	10	95
15	20	80
30	40	60

Based on this information, quality specifications would be established for the product. Acceptable tablets would be required to disintegrate in 3 to 7 minutes and release 50 per cent of their drug content in 4 to 8 minutes under standard laboratory testing conditions. Tablets falling outside this range would be rejected even though they might meet minimum legal standards. This is called "keeping the quality up".

Performance — the ultimate test of product quality — is based on the proven reliability and reproducibility of the dosage form as a drug delivery system. The pharmaceutical new product, in final form, must be tested extensively under controlled clinical conditions to firmly establish its value or efficacy in medicine. Clinical testing — the last phase of proving new product performance — must be done with large numbers of patients. This is a costly, time-consuming, but very necessary operation. Any significant changes in the composition of the product during this last phase would require repeating all or part of the medical testing. In practice, this means that the pharmaceutical development scientist must complete the design of the dosage form and fix its composition two or more years before the product is actually marketed. Designing drug delivery systems that will meet the quality standards of the future presents an enormous challenge to the scientist. Ideally, during the time the product is marketed it should continue to equal or exceed the highest standards. The quality introduced by the designer must endure and must balance with respect to consumer acceptance, reasonable price, manufacturing feasibility, stability and, above all — performance as a drug delivery system.

Appendix

UNITS OF MEASUREMENT, ABBREVIATIONS, AND APPROXIMATE EQUIVALENTS

Length	1 Meter (m.) = 100 centimeters (cm.) = 39.37 inches 1 centimeter (cm.) = 10 millimeters (mm.) 1 Angstrom (A) = 0.00000001 centimeters = 10^{8} cm.
Volume	1 Liter (l.) = 1000 milliliters (ml.) = 1.06 quarts 1 milliliter (ml.) = 1 cubic centimeter (cc.) 30 milliliters (ml.) = 1 fluid ounce.
Weight	1 Kilogram (kg.) = 1000 grams (g.) = 2.2 pounds 1 Gram (g.) = 1000 milligrams (mg.) = 15.43 grains 5 grain aspirin tablet contains 300 milligrams (mg.) aspirin
Temperature	Degrees Centigrade (°C) = 5/9 X (°F - 32) Degrees Kelvin (°K) = °C + 273 Degrees Fahrenheit (°F) = (9/5 X °C) + 32 Room Temperature = 25°C = 77°F

LOGARITHMS, EXPONENTIALS, AND RECIPROCALS

Number	Exponential	Logarithm
10	10^1	1
100	10^2	2
0.01	10^{-2}	-2

Reciprocal Notation

Numbers $1/2 = 2^{-1} = 0.5$

Dimensional Formulas $1/\text{time} = \text{time}^{-1}$

Glossary

Absorption	The passage of drug from the gastro-intestinal tract or from an injection site into the blood.
Adsorption	The adhesion of molecules to the surface of solids.
Ampul	A small, sealed glass vessel for holding a single dose of drug given by hypodermic injection.
Antibiotic	An antibacterial drug produced by a living organism.
Antioxidant	Substance added to prevent or retard destruction of drugs by oxygen.
Applied Research	Experimental studies done mainly to find something useful to man in the immediate or near future.
Availability	The percentage of drug absorbed by the body from a given dose.
Basic Research	Experimental studies done mainly to increase knowledge of the world around us.

Beta Rays	High speed electrons emitted in radioactive disintegrations.
"Blind" Testing	Clinical comparison of a drug dosage form against a placebo (no drug) dosage form, identical in appearance.
Capsule	Tube-like casings made of gelatin for containing a dose of drug.
Chemical Kinetics	Branch of physical chemistry dealing with mathematical description of rates of chemical reactions and prediction of pathways.
Clathrate Compound	A cage-like compound formed by proper match between dimensions of guest molecule and host molecule.
Clinical Testing	Evaluation of dosage forms in human subjects.
Coated Compressed Tablet	A solid dosage form consisting of a compressed tablet coated with sugar.
Complex	A weakly bonded distinct molecular species capable of existing in solution.
Correlation	A relationship between a laboratory test of a dosage form and its clinical performance.
Critical Path	Schedule showing tasks that must be completed in sequence to achieve a development objective.
Crossover Study	Experimental design for a clinical test in which each subject receives each kind of dosage form so that a fair comparison can be made.

Degradation	Loss of drug potency or activity.
Diffusion	Movement of dissolved molecules from a region of high concentration to low.
Disintegration Time	Laboratory test measuring time required for tablet to break up into small granules.
Dissolution Test	Laboratory test to determine amount of drug released from dosage form as a function of time.
Dosage Form	Physical form in which the dose of drug is prepared, e.g. as a tablet or an injection.
Dose	The measured portion of drug to be taken at one time.
Drug Delivery System	Dosage form designed to give efficient and reproducible drug absorption.
Drug Derivative	A drug chemically modified to improve its acceptance, stability or performance.
Drug Metabolite	Compound resulting from chemical transformation of a drug in the body.
Efficacy	Drug effectiveness.
Enteric Coating	Special protective coating applied to tablets which prevents drug release in the acid environment of the stomach but allows release in the mildly alkaline conditions of the intestine.

Enzyme	Complex organic substances such as pepsin that accelerate chemical transformation as in digestion of food.
Ester	An organic compound containing a special linkage between carbon and oxygen atoms $(\text{-}\overset{\overset{\text{O}}{\|}}{\text{C}}\text{-O-})$.
Expiration Dating	Time period that a product will retain not less than 90% of labeled potency.
FDA	The Food and Drug Administration is a U.S. Government agency responsible for enforcing drug laws which require that a drug be safe and effective.
Film-Coated Tablet	Compressed tablet covered with a thin film of water-soluble polymeric material.
Formulation	The specific composition of a dosage form.
Freeze Drying	A process by which solutions are frozen and the water removed under high vacuum so that it passes from solid to gaseous state without becoming liquid.
Granules	Small particles of a solid drug formulation.
Half-Life	Time for a drug blood level to be reduced by one-half.
Hydrolytic Breakdown	Reaction of a drug molecule with water resulting in cleavage into inactive fragments and loss of activity.

Inclusion Compound	A compound formed by a proper match between the dimensions of a guest molecule and host molecule – also known as a Clathrate compound.
Incompatibility	Incapable of being used together because of alteration in the chemical, physical, or biological properties of the drugs.
"Inert" Ingredient	Non-drug component or ingredient of a formulation.
Infusion	A class of fluid products prepared by extracting active principles of a substance with hot water.
Ingredient X	The non-drug components of a formulation.
Intramuscular (I.M.) Injection	Administration of a drug into muscle tissue.
Intravenous (I.V.) Injection	Administration of drug into a vein.
Labeled Drug	Drug containing a radioactive atom as a tracer for testing availability from dosage forms.
Layered-Compressed Tablet	Compressed tablet made by compressing an additional layer onto a previously formed tablet.
LD_{50}	Lethal Dose (50%) is the amount of drug which is fatal to 50 per cent of the experimental animals of a group studied under controlled conditions.

Log Scale Graph	Specially ruled graph paper having distances between horizontal lines marked according to a logarithmic scale.
Mechanism	Detailed information about the steps involved in a chemical reaction.
Molar Concentration	The strength of a solution expressed in Gram-Moles of substance per liter of solution.
Ointment	Semi-solid preparation for external application of drug to the skin.
Ophthalmic Product	Preparation intended for use in the eye.
Oxidation Reaction	Chemical addition of oxygen to a substance.
Parenteral Product	Sterile drug formulations intended to be administered by injection.
pH	A special notation for expressing the concentration of hydrogen ions in a solution; pH is the negative exponent of 10 which gives the hydrogen ion concentration, e.g. pH 7 = 0.0000001 = 1×10^{-7} gram ions per liter.
Pill	A solid, *round* dosage form made by rolling a dough-like mass into tiny spheres or by coating the drug onto sugar spheres in a rolling pan. The term "pill" is often erroneously applied to a compressed tablet.

Physiological Availability	The per cent of dose absorbed from a given dosage form — a measure of efficiency.
Placebo	A dosage form containing *no* drug but identical in appearance, taste, and odor to a drug dosage form.
Plasma	The fluid portion of the blood.
Polymer	Organic compound of high molecular weight composed of repeating structural units. Polymers are often called "plastics."
Potency	Activity or effectiveness of the drug contained in a dosage form.
Press-Coated Tablet	Tablet prepared by compressing a coating onto a previously formed tablet.
Prolonged Action Tablet	Dosage form designed to provide an extended period of action for a given drug.
Pyrogens	Waste materials produced during the growth of microorganisms which can cause fever if injected into a man.
Quality Control	An organized effort to control the quality in the formulation, manufacture, and distribution of a pharmaceutical product.
Reactive Compound	Organic radicals possessing an unpaired electron; they are capable of interacting with molecules to release additional radicals and thereby cause a chain reaction.

Scale-up Studies	Process of making larger quantities of an experimental product in stepwise progression from small laboratory batches to full scale production batches.
Sequestering Agent	Compound capable of binding or de-activating metal ions in solution.
Shelf-Life	Time period a product will retain at least 90 per cent of potency indicated on its label.
Stability	Resistance of a drug to deterioration or loss of potency.
Sterile Products	Dosage forms that are free from micro-organisms, e.g., products administered by hypodermic injection.
Subcutaneous (Sub Q.) Injection	Administration of drug immediately beneath the skin.
Sugar-Coated Tablet	Compressed tablets covered with a sugar coating.
Sustained Release Product	Dosage form designed to provide an extended period of action for a given drug.
Surfactant	Substance causing reduction in surface tension. Familiar examples include soaps and synthetic detergents.
Synthetic Drugs	Drug compounds made by chemical synthesis.
Tablet	Solid dosage form made by compressing a mixture of drug in combination with special ingredients.

Tincture	A fluid dosage form consisting of a water-alcohol solution of medicinal substances.
Topical Products	Dosage forms designed to be applied to skin or mucous membranes.
Toxicology Data	Information about the safety of a drug and its dosage forms.
Tristimulus Concept	Description of a color in terms of hue, purity, and lightness.
Viscosity	Resistance offered by a fluid to flow.
Wetting Agent	Substance which lowers surface tension of a solution and facilitates penetration of water into pores and voids of solids.

Subject Index